The Natural PHARMACIST™ TNP.com

Inside—Find the Answers to These Questions and More

☑ Can garlic help lower my elevated cholesterol levels? (See page 19.)

☑ Will it reduce high blood pressure? (See page 30.)

☑ Is one form of garlic more effective than another? (See page 42.)

☑ How much should I take? (See page 48.)

☑ Are there any side effects? (See page 54.)

☑ Can taking garlic help prevent heart attacks? (See page 37.)

☑ What medications should I not combine with garlic? (See page 61.)

☑ How effective is red yeast rice for lowering my cholesterol? (See page 65.)

☑ What are the benefits and risks of niacin? (See page 81.)

☑ Which foods can lower cholesterol? (See page 92.)

THE NATURAL PHARMACIST™ Library

Feverfew and Migraines

Heart Disease Prevention

Kava and Anxiety

Natural Health Bible

Natural Treatments for Arthritis

Natural Treatments for Colds and Flus

Natural Treatments for Diabetes

Natural Treatments for High Cholesterol

Natural Treatments to Improve Memory

Natural Treatments for Menopause

PMS

Reducing Cancer Risk

Saw Palmetto and the Prostate

St. John's Wort and Depression

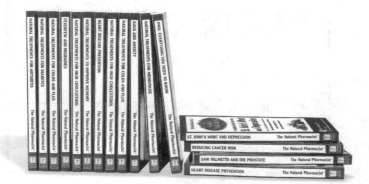

To order, visit www.TNP.com

Natural Treatments for High Cholesterol

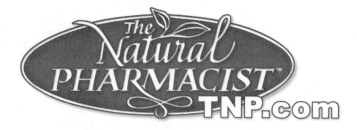

Natural Treatments for High Cholesterol

Darin Ingels, N.D.

Series Editors

Steven Bratman, M.D.

David Kroll, Ph.D.

A DIVISION OF PRIMA PUBLISHING

3000 Lava Ridge Court ■ Roseville, California 95661

(800) 632-8676 ■ www.TNP.com

Published in association with TNP.com.

Warning—Disclaimer
This book is not intended to provide medical advice and is sold with the understanding that the publisher and the author are not liable for the misconception or misuse of information provided. The author and Prima Publishing shall have neither liability nor responsibility to any person or entity with respect to any loss, damage, or injury caused or alleged to be caused directly or indirectly by the information contained in this book or the use of any products mentioned. Readers should not use any of the products discussed in this book without the advice of a medical professional.

TNP.COM, THENATURALPHARMACIST.COM, THE NATURAL PHARMACIST, and PRIMA HEALTH are trademarks of Prima Communications Inc. The Prima colophon is a trademark of Prima Communications Inc., registered with the United States Patent and Trademark Office.

The Food and Drug Administration has not approved the use of any of the natural treatments discussed in this book. This book, and the information contained herein, has not been approved by the Food and Drug Administration.

Pseudonyms have been used throughout to protect the privacy of the individuals involved.

All products mentioned in this book are trademarks of their respective companies.

Illustrations by Helene Stevens and Gale Mueller. Illustrations © 1999 by Prima Publishing. All rights reserved.

Library of Congress Cataloging-in-Publication Data
Ingels, Darin.
    Natural treatments for high cholesterol / Darin Ingels.
      p. cm.—(The natural pharmacist)
    Includes bibliographical references and index.
    ISBN 0-7615-2467-3
    1. Hypercholesteremia—Diet Therapy. 2. Garlic—Therapeutic use.
    3. Atherosclerosis—Diet therapy. I. Title. II. Series.
    RG632.H83I54   1999
    616.1'2305—dc21   98—50707
                                                            CIP

00 01 02 03 HH 10 9 8 7 6 5 4 3 2 1
Printed in the United States of America

How to Order
Single copies may be ordered from Prima Publishing, 3000 Lava Ridge Court, Roseville, CA 95661; telephone (800) 632-8676. Quantity discounts are also available. On your letterhead, include information concerning the intended use of the books and the number of books you wish to purchase.

Visit us online at www.TNP.com and www.primahealth.com

*Special thanks to Drs. Brammer,
Dipasquale, Lamden, and Donovan,
Jon Goodman, Melissa Macfarlane,
Susie Wickstead, my families,
and especially my wife, Michelle,
for her love and support.*

Contents

What Makes This Book Different?   xi

Introduction   xv

1. Atherosclerosis and High Cholesterol   1

2. Garlic for High Cholesterol   11

3. Other Supplements for High Cholesterol   65

4. Niacin and High Cholesterol   81

5. Lifestyle Changes   91

6. Conventional Treatments for High Cholesterol   101

7. Putting It All Together   111

Notes   115

Index   129

About the Author and Series Editors   139

What Makes This Book Different?

The interest in natural medicine has never been greater. According to the National Association of Chain Drug Stores, 65 million Americans are using natural supplements, and the number is growing! Yet, it is hard for the consumer to find trustworthy sources for balanced information about this emerging field. Why? Frankly, natural medicine has had a checkered history. From snake oil potions sold at the turn of the century to those books, magazines, and product catalogs that hype miracle cures today, this is a field where exaggerated claims have been the norm. Proponents of natural medicine have tended to abuse science, treating it more as a marketing tool than a means of discovering the truth.

But there is truth to be found. Studies of vitamins, minerals, and other food supplements have been with us since these nutritional substances were first discovered, and the level and quality of this science has grown dramatically in the last 20 years. Herbal medicine has been neglected in the United States, but in Europe, this, the oldest of all healing arts, has been the subject of tremendous and ongoing scientific interest.

At present, for a number of herbs and supplements, it is possible to give reasonably scientific answers to the questions: How well does this work? How safe is it? What types of conditions is it best used for?

THE NATURAL PHARMACIST series is designed to cut through the hype and tell you what is known and what remains to be scientifically proven regarding popular natural treatments. These books are more conservative than any others available, more honest about the weaknesses of natural approaches, more fair in their comparisons of natural and conventional treatments. You won't find any miracle cures here, but you will discover useful options that can help you become healthier.

Why Choose Natural Treatments?

Although the science behind natural medicine continues to grow, this is still a much less scientifically validated field than conventional medicine. You might ask, "Why should I resort to an herb that is only partly proven, when I could take a drug with solid science behind it?" There are at least three good reasons to consider natural alternatives.

First, some herbs and supplements offer benefits that are not matched by any conventional drug. Vitamin E is a good example. It appears to help prevent prostate cancer, a benefit that no standard medication can claim. Also, vitamin E almost certainly helps prevent heart disease. While there are standard drugs that also prevent heart disease, vitamin E works differently and may be able to complement many of the other approaches.

Another example is the herb milk thistle. Studies strongly suggest that this herb can protect the liver from injury. There is no pill or tablet your doctor can prescribe to do the same.

Even if the science behind some of these treatments is less than perfect, when the risks are low and the possible benefit high, a natural treatment may be worth trying. It is a little-known fact that for many conventional treatments the science is less than perfect as well, and physicians must balance uncertain benefits against incompletely understood risks.

A second reason to consider natural therapies is that some may offer benefits comparable to those of drugs with fewer side effects. The herb St. John's wort is a good example. Reasonably strong scientific evidence suggests that this herb is an effective treatment for mild to moderate depression, while producing fewer side effects on average than conventional medications. Saw palmetto for benign enlargement of the prostate, ginkgo for relieving symptoms and perhaps slowing the progression of Alzheimer's disease, and glucosamine for osteoarthritis are other examples. This is not to say that herbs and supplements are completely harmless—they're not—but for most the level of risk is quite low.

Finally, there is a philosophical point to consider. For many people, it "feels" better to use a treatment that comes from nature instead of from a laboratory. Just as you might rather wear all-cotton clothing than polyester, or look at a mountain landscape rather than the skyscrapers of a downtown city, natural treatments may simply feel more compatible with your view of life. We can quibble endlessly about just what "natural" means and whether a certain treatment is "actually" natural or not, but such arguments are beside the point. The difference is in the feeling, and feelings matter. In fact, having a good feeling about taking an herb may lead you to use it more consistently than you would a prescription drug.

Of course, at times synthetic drugs may be necessary and even lifesaving. But on many other occasions it may be quite reasonable to turn to an herb or supplement instead of a drug.

To make good decisions you need good information. Unfortunately, while hundreds of books on alternative medicine are published every year, many are highly misleading. The phrase "studies prove" is often used when the studies in question are so small or so badly conducted that they prove nothing at all. You may even find that the "data" from other books comes from studies with petri dishes and not real people!

You can't even assume that books written by well-known authors are scientifically sound. Many of these authors rely on secondary writers, leading to a game of "telephone," where misconceptions are passed around from book to book. And there's a strong tendency to exaggerate the power of natural remedies, whitewashing them with selective reporting.

THE NATURAL PHARMACIST series gives you the balanced information you need to make informed decisions about your health needs. Setting a new, high standard of accuracy and objectivity, these books take a realistic look at the herbs and supplements you read about in the news. You will encounter both favorable and unfavorable studies in these pages and will learn about both the benefits and the risks of natural treatments.

THE NATURAL PHARMACIST series is the source you can trust.

Steven Bratman, M.D.
David Kroll, Ph.D.

Introduction

If you asked most people on the street what the greatest health concern facing America is right now, you might get answers such as "cancer" or "AIDS." What many don't realize is cardiovascular disease is the number one killer in the developed world. In America alone, over 58 million people suffer from such problems as angina, heart attacks, strokes, and aortic aneurysm, and almost 1 million die each year as a consequence.

While there are many causes of cardiovascular disease, high cholesterol is undoubtedly one of the most important. Unfortunately, high cholesterol by itself does not usually cause symptoms. In fact, the symptoms may not become apparent until the onset of crushing chest pain, and the arrival of an ambulance to take you to intensive care. This is one disease that you must identify early, to spare yourself avoidable risk and suffering.

Interestingly, physicians did not at first realize that high cholesterol levels were cause for concern. Actually, for a while, they thought low cholesterol was the cause of heart attacks. (This misconception came about because right after a heart attack, the measured cholesterol level is unusually low.) The breakthrough came after the residents of Framingham, Massachusetts, agreed to participate in an enormous long-term study that continues to the present day. It was this Framingham study that woke up the medical world to the risks presented by high cholesterol levels in the blood. Because of Framingham, by the late 1950s, we could no longer eat a breakfast consisting of sausage, bacon, eggs fried in lard, and white toast liberally smeared with butter without imagining clumps of fat sticking to our arteries. The low-fat movement had begun.

Besides dietary changes, medical researchers began to search for treatments that could reduce cholesterol levels. The vitamin niacin was one of the earliest successful treatments, and is now so well established it has become a conventional treatment. In the 1980s, an advanced type of drug called HMG-CoA reductase inhibitors became available. These drugs were capable of specifically reducing cholesterol production with relatively few side effects.

Another approach to high cholesterol was pursued by researchers in Germany over the same time period: They investigated the potential benefits of the natural herb garlic. As far back as ancient Roman times, garlic was said to "clear the arteries." Modern research has discovered that this antiquated belief has a basis in science. Although the evidence is not yet definitive, it does appear that appropriate use of garlic can significantly reduce cholesterol levels, and it may also help prevent strokes and heart attacks.

Soy foods have recently been permitted by the FDA to boast a "heart-healthy" label for their cholesterol-lowering benefits. Gugulipid, red yeast rice, pantethine, tocotrienols, fish oil, aortic glycosaminoglycans, and carnitine are other promising options.

While most of these treatments appear to be fairly safe, there are some potential risks that need to be considered. This book will tell you everything you need to know about these natural options for high cholesterol.

Natural Treatments for High Cholesterol

Atherosclerosis and High Cholesterol

T here is only one reason why you would want to lower your cholesterol when it is high: elevated cholesterol levels cause atherosclerosis. In turn, atherosclerosis leads to two of the major causes of death in the developed world: heart disease and strokes. This chapter discusses atherosclerosis and its relationship to cholesterol levels.

Atherosclerosis is a disorder of the larger arteries in the body that leads to thickening and hardening of the arterial wall, and deposits of a fatty substance known as *plaque*. It is the leading cause of death in men over the age of 35 and of all people over the age of 45. Atherosclerosis and its related diseases cause approximately 50% of all deaths in the United States.[1]

Atherosclerosis in the coronary arteries of the heart diminishes the flow of blood to the heart muscle (see figure 1) causing a type of pain known as *angina*. Blood clots also tend to form along the walls of the arteries in the heart. The clots may break free and lodge themselves across the width of the vessel, completely blocking the flow of blood. The part of the heart muscle that is fed by that artery then dies from lack of oxygen. Such blockage of the artery is commonly called a heart attack. (A similar process can occur in the blood vessels that feed the brain, leading to a stroke.)

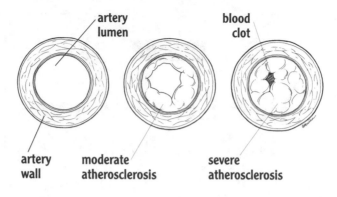

Figure 1. *Cross-section of three coronary arteries*

Atherosclerosis can also weaken the wall of a major artery, causing it to enlarge (becoming an aneurysm), leak blood, and eventually rupture. Atherosclerosis in the arteries of the legs causes pain with mild exercise, a condition known as *intermittent claudication.* Other consequences of atherosclerosis include kidney disease and impotence.

Obviously, atherosclerosis is a disease that requires serious medical attention; left untreated its consequences are serious. The good news is that atherosclerosis can be prevented and—even better—there is reasonably good evidence that it can even be *reversed* by eliminating the factors that cause it.

Risk Factors for Atherosclerosis

In 1948, a historic medical research project began. Known as the Framingham Heart Study, it aimed to follow the lives of 5,209 people living in Framingham, Massachusetts, for 30 years. The results have led to major changes in the lifestyles of many Americans and people all over the world. The Framingham study forever changed our view of food, turning the once-innocent pleasure of a breakfast of bacon and eggs, coffee with cream, and thickly buttered toast into a dangerous luxury.

The Framingham researchers found four major risk factors for atherosclerosis: high cholesterol in the blood, cigarette smoking, high blood pressure, and diabetes. Other probable risk factors include a sedentary lifestyle, a diet high in animal fats, being male, a family history of early heart disease, and high blood levels of homocysteine. (Homocysteine is a chemical in the blood that appears to be a major risk factor for heart disease.)

The following chapters primarily address the first of these risk factors—high cholesterol levels in the blood. For more detailed information about the other risk factors, see *The Natural Pharmacist: Heart Disease Prevention.*

What Causes Atherosclerosis?

Despite decades of intensive study, we still do not fully understand the causes of atherosclerosis, although we do know a great deal. Contrary to popular belief, cholesterol doesn't simply accumulate in arteries the way grease builds up in pipes. Rather, the process involves progressive damage to the lining of arteries, in which cholesterol plays only a contributing role.

Although symptoms don't appear until adulthood, atherosclerosis comes on slowly, beginning early in childhood and only gradually progressing to full-scale disease. Several studies have shown that signs of atherosclerosis can be found in children as young as 1 year old, and that by age 10 almost all children have fatty streaks in their blood vessels.[2,3]

When plaque restricts the flow of blood, symptoms such as angina, intermittent claudication, and temporary strokes (called TIAs) can result.

Fatty streaks are flat, yellow spots in the artery wall, which can grow up to 1 centimeter or longer. Because they are flat, fatty streaks don't obstruct the blood vessel or disrupt blood flow. However, over time they can gradually develop into full-scale atherosclerosis. The leading theory regarding how this occurs is the "response to injury" hypothesis. According to this theory, atherosclerosis is first triggered by an injury to the inner lining of the arterial wall (the *endothelium*).

According to the American Heart Association, as many as 97 million Americans have elevated blood cholesterol levels, with almost 38 million adults exceeding levels defined as "high risk."

What can cause such an injury? The endothelium can be injured by direct physical strain, such as high blood pressure. Also, irritating substances circulating in the blood can cause damage. Some of the suspected irritants in the blood include low-density lipoprotein molecules (also called LDL or "bad" cholesterol), homocysteine, glucose, and free radicals. Atherosclerosis tends to develop especially quickly at forks in the blood vessels, probably because the current of blood strikes those areas with particular force.

Once the endothelium has been damaged, a type of white blood cell adheres to the site of injury, then works its way deeper into the arterial wall. There, it is transformed into a scavenger cell called a *macrophage*. Macrophages collect molecules of cholesterol and other fatty substances until they are so fat-filled they look like microscopic fatty snowballs. At the same time, platelets (cells that normally circulate in the bloodstream waiting to repair leaks in blood vessels) begin to stick to the damaged artery wall and form a plug. When they do this, they also release several chemicals that cause muscle cells to migrate to the area. These muscle cells then reproduce, yielding fibrous substances and thickening the fatty streak.

Over time, more white blood cells arrive, and a growing collection of dead cells, fat, calcium, and fibrous tissue makes the artery wall swell. Eventually, the swelling reaches a size where it is called a *fibrous plaque*. Individual fibrous plaques subsequently connect to form what is called *complicated plaque*. Complicated plaque continues to grow in both size and thickness until the *lumen* (open space) of the artery becomes partially or completely blocked, or until the artery wall becomes so weak that it ruptures. Pieces of plaque can also break free from the vessel wall, creating small bleeding spots. The body responds by forming a blood clot to stop the bleeding. Clots may also form simply because the plaque's surface is ragged. Such *thrombi*, as the clots are called, can become integrated into the plaque or, even worse, break off and completely obstruct the artery somewhere downstream. Broken off bits of plaque can also do this.

When plaque narrows the open space in the blood vessel and restricts the flow of blood, symptoms such as angina, intermittent claudication, and temporary strokes called *transient ischemic attacks* (TIAs) can result. However, outright blockage of the blood vessel by a blood clot or a piece of plaque can lead to full-blown strokes and heart attacks.

The Link Between High Cholesterol and Atherosclerosis

Although cholesterol doesn't clog arteries directly, there is absolutely no doubt that high cholesterol is a major cause of atherosclerosis. In the Framingham and other large studies, elevated levels of blood cholesterol have been associated with as much as a 300% increase in the rate of death due to heart attacks. The higher the blood cholesterol levels, the greater the heart attack rate. Furthermore, in animal studies where high levels of cholesterol were induced, atherosclerosis has been found to develop at a greatly increased rate.

According to the American Heart Association, as many as 97 million Americans have elevated blood cholesterol levels, with almost 38 million adults exceeding levels defined as "high risk." Clearly, controlling your cholesterol level is one of the most important health-affirming steps you can take.

What Is Cholesterol?

Cholesterol is a kind of *lipid,* or fat, in the body. Although cholesterol plays a role in atherosclerosis, it is also an essential substance in the body. The body uses it to make bile, which it uses to digest fats, as well as to produce vitamin D and hormones such as estrogen, progesterone, and testosterone.

The body directly manufactures about two-thirds of its total cholesterol. The other third comes into the body through food, primarily from animal products such as meat, milk, and eggs. Most cells in the body can make cholesterol, but more than 90% is created in the liver and the walls of the intestine.

Lipoproteins: "Good" Cholesterol Versus "Bad" Cholesterol

As a fat, cholesterol isn't water soluble, so it doesn't dissolve in the blood. To allow it to move around the body, a special carrier molecule known as a *lipoprotein* attaches to it. Lipoproteins have the capacity to help fats dissolve in water. They shuttle cholesterol and triglycerides between the different tissues of the body. (See How Do You Know If You Have High Cholesterol?) There are several different types of lipoprotein/cholesterol packages, and each has its own effect on the body. The major types are called low-density lipoprotein (LDL), high-density lipoprotein (HDL), and very low-density lipoprotein (VLDL). LDL appears to be the most harmful type and, therefore, is often referred to as "bad" cholesterol. Studies show that higher LDL levels are directly associated with accelerated atherosclerosis. Conversely, HDL is regarded as the "good" cholesterol, because higher levels of it are associated with a lower incidence of atherosclerosis. HDL's job appears to be carrying cholesterol from the tissues back to the liver for redistribution or elimination. There is some evidence that garlic can specifically reduce LDL levels and raise HDL levels.

A special form of LDL called lipoprotein(a) may be even more harmful than regular LDL.[4,5] High levels of lipoprotein(a) have been associated with a tenfold increase in the risk for heart disease, regardless of total cholesterol and LDL levels. Lipoprotein(a) contains an additional protein that increases its ability to stick to the artery wall, apparently increasing its capacity to cause damage.

If HDL (high-density lipoprotein) is "good" cholesterol and LDL (low-density lipoprotein) is "bad" cholesterol, one would think that VLDL (very low-density lipoprotein) is "very bad" cholesterol. However, this isn't the case. Here's why: Instead of cholesterol, VLDL primarily contains other fatty substances called *triglycerides.* Triglycerides are not as harmful as cholesterol, although they too may accelerate atherosclerosis.

How Do You Know If You Have High Cholesterol?

Your doctor can determine your total blood cholesterol, HDL, and triglyceride levels with a blood test called a *lipid profile.* A mathematical calculation can then determine your LDL level as well. (VLDL levels are not usually reported, because total blood triglyceride levels are more relevant.) Because a fatty or high cholesterol meal can temporarily raise your cholesterol level, you need to get your blood drawn for a lipid profile in the morning before you've eaten.

The United States' National Cholesterol Education Program currently recommends a goal of total cholesterol below 200 mg/dL (milligrams per deciliter). Total cholesterol levels between 200 and 240 mg/dL are considered to be borderline high; levels above 240 mg/dL are considered high

Studies have shown that for every 1% drop in total cholesterol there is a 2% decrease in the risk of having a heart attack.

risk. These levels are important not only as indicators of risk of heart disease, but also as a guideline to help you and your doctor choose among available therapies. Optimally, LDL ("bad"

Dave's Story

Dave, a 26-year-old man, was concerned about his weight. Although he didn't look obese, Dave was about 25 pounds overweight for his height. Dave's father had died of a heart attack at a young age and his grandfather had also died young as a result of a stroke. Dave worked long hours as a computer analyst, so he only had the chance to eat one meal a day (which was always fast food), and he rarely exercised. Along with these risk factors for heart disease (sedentary lifestyle, high-fat diet, and family history), his total cholesterol was 256 mg/dL (too high), his LDL cholesterol was 151 mg/dL (also too high), and his HDL was 25 mg/dL (too low). His blood pressure was normal.

cholesterol) levels should be below 130 mg/dL, and HDL ("good" cholesterol) levels should be greater than 30 mg/dL. Triglyceride levels should be less than 250 mg/dL, and lipoprotein(a) levels should ideally fall below 20 mg/dL.

Another useful piece of information for determining your risk is the ratio between your total cholesterol level and HDL level, as well as the ratio between your HDL and LDL levels. These ratios are often called *cardiac risk factors* because they too relate to your risk of heart disease. The total cholesterol-to-HDL ratio should be no greater than 4.5:1, and the LDL-to-HDL ratio should not exceed 2.5:1. Higher ratios indicate a moderate to high risk, with the risk increasing as the ratio increases.

These values and ratios are tools that you and your doctor can use to assess your risk for atherosclerosis and cardiovascular disease. Studies have shown that for every 1% drop in total cholesterol there is a 2% decrease in the risk of having a heart attack. The risk for heart attack drops even more—by as much as 4%—when HDL levels increase by 1%.

He improved his diet and increased his level of exercise, and he began to take a standardized garlic supplement that contained the equivalent of 4,000 mg of fresh garlic daily. (See How to Take Garlic in chapter 2 for more information on standardized supplements.) After 3 months on this program, he had dropped almost 15 pounds, and he said that he felt great. His total cholesterol had fallen to 206 mg/dL, his LDL cholesterol had dropped to 122 mg/dL, and his HDL cholesterol had risen to 35 mg/dL. It was a dramatic improvement.

Which helped most, the lifestyle changes or the garlic? It's hard to say. See The Scientific Evidence in chapter 2 for information that suggests garlic can have a positive impact on lipid levels.

How Do You Know If You Have Atherosclerosis?

A major problem in diagnosing atherosclerosis is that there are usually no symptoms until it is fairly advanced. In the arteries of the heart, blockage can reach up to 90% before you begin to feel chest pain. Sometimes with a stethoscope, it is possible to hear a sound made by blood passing through a narrowed artery. This sound, technically called a *bruit* (pronounced BREW-ee), is usually medium-pitched, with a blowing quality to it. A physician can also feel for a vibration called a *thrill.* However, you really want to catch atherosclerosis before it reaches this point. If your doctor suspects you have a significant amount of atherosclerosis, there are several technologically advanced tools that can reveal how much blockage has occurred.

A major problem in diagnosing atherosclerosis is that there are usually no symptoms until it is fairly advanced.

Diagnostic imaging such as Doppler studies (similar to the Doppler radar used for weather forecasting), catheterization, x-ray, and CT scans may be used, depending on which particular arteries are affected and the type of information your doctor wants. Obviously, the best plan is to assess your risk factors for atherosclerosis and to get examined now rather than waiting until the condition has set in.

Garlic for
High Cholesterol

I s it an herb or a food? Garlic *(Allium sativum)* has been used as both a food and medicine by cultures world-wide for more than 5,000 years. A familiar sight at the grocery store (where you can find whole garlic, garlic powder, garlic salt, and pickled and minced garlic), garlic is also one of the most widely prescribed medicinal herbs today. In Germany it's considered one of the best all-around heart herbs because of its apparent effects on cholesterol, blood pressure, free radicals, and blood clotting.

What we think of as garlic is actually the base of the garlic plant, also known as the *bulb.* Each bulb, or head, of garlic contains a number of separate *cloves.* Each clove is wrapped in a papery sheath, which must be peeled away before the garlic can be used. The garlic bulb itself is also wrapped in thin, papery layers of white or reddish-white plant material. (See figure 2.)

A staple in many home gardens, garlic is relatively easy to cultivate. If you've grown garlic in your garden, you know that the garlic plant includes a long, smooth stem that rises up to 3 feet from the ground. Like its cousin, the leek, the garlic plant produces several long, thin, sharply tapered leaves that originate close to the ground. The garlic bulb grows just beneath the

Visit Us at TNP.com

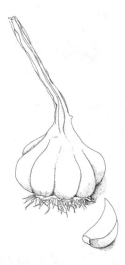

Figure 2. *Garlic*

ground, and when mature, it often pokes through the soil at the base of the stem.

In the summer, a cluster of purple-white flowers encased in a paper-thin sheath appears at the top of the stem. If you look closely among the flowers, you will see what look like 20 to 30 tiny bulbs. These *bulbils* are parts of the plant that can be used to grow more garlic. However, the quickest way to grow good-size garlic is to plant a single clove you want to harvest.

Why Is It Called Garlic?

"Garlic" is derived from the Anglo-Saxon word *garleac,* meaning "spear-leek"—an apt description of the plant's general appearance and the slender, hard stem that resembles its cousin, the leek. The Latin name for garlic is *Allium sativum. Allium* is the Latin word for garlic, and according to some, it is derived from a Celtic word meaning "hot" or "sharp taste." Others believe that it is derived from a Latin word meaning "to smell." Most people would agree that either term describes garlic's characteristic strong odor and sharp, hot taste.

Sativum simply means "cultivated." Garlic has been cultivated since the beginning of recorded history, and its survival attests to humanity's great love for this herb. In fact, garlic has been cultivated for so long that it no longer grows in the wild, although other *Allium* species do.

What Is in Garlic?

Garlic gets much of its strong odor from sulfur. The herb contains a considerable amount of sulfur, in the form of several different chemical compounds. Garlic's major sulfur-containing ingredient, *alliin*, is relatively odorless. However, crushing or cutting garlic brings an enzyme called *allinase* into contact with alliin, producing a powerfully aromatic substance called *allicin*.

Garlic has been used as both a food and medicine by cultures worldwide for more than 5,000 years.

You can see (or rather, *smell*) this chemical reaction at work with this simple experiment: Carefully peel a clove of fresh garlic, without scraping or cutting into the clove. Sniff the clove. Then smash it with the flat part of a knife and sniff again. The powerful odor released after the clove has been smashed lets you know that alliin and allinase have combined to produce allicin.

In addition to giving garlic most of its strong odor, allicin can blister the skin and kill bacteria, viruses, and fungi. Presumably, the garlic plant uses allicin and other sulfur compounds to protect itself from harmful microbes and insects. Allicin also appears to be at least partly responsible for garlic's medicinal effects.

Many researchers, in fact, believe that allicin is garlic's primary active ingredient. This is because laboratory research has found that allicin chemically inhibits enzymes responsible for making cholesterol. Furthermore, some garlic products that do not contain alliin have not proven effective in clinical studies. Other experts, however, disagree with the belief that allicin is the primary active ingredient. For more information, see The Scientific Evidence later in this chapter.

Allicin quickly breaks down into other chemical compounds that may also contribute to garlic's medicinal properties. One of the challenges for manufacturers in the medicinal preparation of garlic is to ensure that either allicin itself or alliin ready to be converted into allicin (and other chemicals) remains in the finished product.

Garlic also contains many chemical compounds that do not include sulfur. These compounds include several B vitamins, minerals, flavonoids, various amino acids, proteins, lipids, steroids, and 12 trace elements. These compounds contribute to the growth and life of the garlic plant, but we don't know whether they play a role in lowering cholesterol.

What Was Garlic Used for Historically?

Botanists generally believe that garlic originated somewhere in central Asia, because other species of *Allium* have been found growing in the wild in an area near the borders of southern Russia and western China. This area has always been a major passageway between Asia and Europe, which may explain how garlic became distributed throughout the world.

The earliest written account of garlic appears on Sumerian clay tablets dating from around 2600 B.C. Inscriptions on these tablets describe the culinary and medicinal uses of garlic, suggesting its use in warding off disease and improving health. The Assyrians, whose civilization followed that of the Sumerians, described similar uses of garlic and used it to treat infections, diarrhea, and inflammation.

An even earlier historical reference to garlic can be found in relics from ancient Egypt. Clay models of garlic were discovered in the tomb of El Mahasna, who died circa 3750 B.C. Similar clay models, as well as actual bulbs of dried garlic, were common in Egyptian tombs, including the tomb of Pharaoh Tutankhamen ("King Tut"). We don't know for certain why the ancient Egyptians felt so strongly about garlic that they would involve it in burial ceremonies, but later, ancient Greeks and Romans wrote that they believed the Egyptians regarded garlic as sacred.

One of the most interesting references to garlic appears in an ancient Egyptian papyrus document known as the Ebers Codex, which was written circa 1550 B.C. The Codex lists more than 880 remedies used at that time; 22 of those references involved garlic. Another Egyptian papyrus from around the same time describes how the men who were working on the pyramids revolted because their daily rations of garlic, radishes, and onions were cut back. The workers apparently believed that garlic gave them strength and protected them from disease.

> **The earliest known historical reference to garlic was in ancient Egypt. Clay models of garlic were discovered in the tomb of El Mahasna, who died circa 3750 B.C.**

The ancient Greek historian Herodotus, who traveled through Egypt around 450 B.C., described inscriptions on the walls of the Great Pyramid detailing the quantity of garlic, radishes, and onions consumed by the workers—another sign that the ancient Egyptians took garlic very seriously.

While the Israelites lived in Egypt, they too came to use garlic as a staple food. The Bible tells how the Hebrews, after escaping their captivity in Egypt, still had fond memories of Egyptian garlic.

An old Jewish tradition holds that eating garlic on the eve of the Sabbath will encourage matrimonial lovemaking. Medical traditions in India also ascribe aphrodisiac powers to garlic.

The early Greek and Roman physicians Hippocrates, Dioscorides, Pliny the Elder, and Galen wrote of garlic's healing properties. Hippocrates, the father of medicine, recommended garlic for infections, wounds, leprosy, cancer, and digestive disorders. He was also the first to comment on garlic's possible side effects. Among these, Hippocrates noted, were the aggravation of various types of pain and increased urine flow.

> Then . . . the Sons of Israel began to wail again, "Who will give us meat to eat?" They said, "Think of the fish we used to eat free in Egypt, the cucumbers, melons, leeks, onions and garlic. Here we are, wasting away, stripped of everything, there is nothing but manna for us to look at."
> (Numbers 11:4–6)

Dioscorides lived in the first century A.D. and is known today as the father of pharmacy. He created a type of herbal catalog called a *materia medica.* A *materia medica* lists not only the herbs, but also their known or suspected medicinal properties, how to identify the herbs, and where to find them. In his *materia medica,* Dioscorides said that garlic was used to treat the bites of rabid dogs as well as chronic coughs, painful teeth, and—impressively, given what we know today—"to clear the arteries." Galen, the leading physician of Roman times, called garlic *theriaca rusticorum,* or "peasants' heal-all," as a testament to garlic's reputation as an effective folk treatment for many diseases. This term carried over into the Middle Ages, where it became known as Poor Man's Theriacle (*theriaca* is Latin for "antidote") due to the townspeople's widespread use of garlic to treat numerous common illnesses. This was later changed to Poor Man's Treacle.

Garlic has also been well used in traditional Chinese medicine. *Da suan,* as it is called in Chinese, was first described in writing around A.D. 500. The Chinese used garlic to treat dysentery, colds, parasites, coughs, and poisoning. Today, it is still used in some traditional Chinese herbal formulas for similar conditions.

The most infamous use of garlic arose in the early eighteenth century in Marseilles, France. Bubonic plague was raging through the city. Although most criminals were too afraid of catching the plague to rob the houses of the ailing, one small band of thieves fearlessly looted the city and robbed the sick and dead. When one of the thieves was finally caught, he testified that he and his cohorts had been consuming garlic soaked in wine and vinegar, and also covering their clothes and bodies in the mixture. The story of their defense against the plague soon swept the countryside and became a popular treatment for preventing illness. This concoction, which became known as Four Thieves Vinegar, is still sold in France—although today it's used as a seasoning rather than to ward off the Black Death.

In more recent history, World War I doctors used fresh garlic as a poultice applied to the wounds of injured soldiers to prevent infection. The British government was so impressed with the results that it encouraged the public to produce as many bulbs as possible, offering a handsome fee for providing the natural antibiotic. When World War II began, antibiotics had started to replace garlic. However, countries that couldn't get enough antibiotics continued to use the herb, which led to garlic becoming known as Russian penicillin.

After World War II, penicillin and other new antibiotics rapidly displaced garlic in American medicine. Two pharmaceutical companies continued to manufacture garlic preparations for intestinal spasms and hypertension, but these drugs were discontinued by 1950, and garlic disappeared from almost every physician's medical bag.

However, European physicians continued to research garlic's medicinal properties. With the development of effective antibiotics, interest in garlic shifted from its antibacterial effects to its influence on cholesterol. As you

Sales of garlic supplements in the United States have more than doubled since the early 1990s.

will learn, garlic is regaining popularity in the United States as well as in Europe as a medicinal herb, and there is strong evidence that it can be effective in reducing cholesterol levels (see The Scientific Evidence). In fact, sales of garlic supplements in the United States have more than doubled since the early 1990s.

Garlic and Modern Medicine

Germany's Commission E is an official governmental agency that performs a job similar to that of the U.S. Food and Drug Administration (FDA), only it's specifically focused on herbs. In 1988 the commission authorized the use of garlic preparations "as an adjunct to dietary measures in patients with elevated blood lipids and for the prevention of age-related vascular changes." Stated simply, garlic is used to lower cholesterol and prevent hardening of the arteries.

> **Today, garlic's primary modern use is to lower cholesterol and prevent hardening of the arteries.**

Garlic may also have a beneficial effect on high blood pressure, although the evidence is not as strong as it is for lowering cholesterol. Studies further suggest that garlic may "thin" the blood and help prevent blood clots. Finally, garlic possesses antioxidant properties similar to those of vitamin E and vitamin C. These potential benefits may enhance the herb's power against atherosclerosis (hardening of the arteries) by attacking the disease from a different direction. This subject is discussed in greater depth in The Scientific Evidence and Beyond Cholesterol: Garlic's Other Potential Benefits for Your Arteries. Regular use of garlic has also been associated with a reduction in the incidence of cancer.[1,2]

As mentioned, the most common historical use of garlic was for the treatment and prevention of infections. However, according to a modern German text on herbs, "the antimicrobial properties of garlic are mainly of historical interest, and have no practical significance for treatment of infectious diseases today."[3] There is no evidence that garlic is an effective antibiotic or antifungal drug when taken internally. However, garlic does appear to fight bacteria and fungi when you apply it directly to the skin.[4] But you have to be careful using it this way, as garlic can cause blisters.

The Scientific Evidence

If you have read a magazine or watched television lately, you have probably noticed an ad or two telling you how herbs are going to change your life. Unfortunately, many of the claims made for herbs are more marketing hype than anything else. Herbal medicines are not miraculous cure-alls. Like all medicines, they have varying results for different people.

Well-designed scientific studies are the only way to sort the hype from the reality. Unfortunately, this kind of research has lagged behind for herbs, especially in the United States. Nonetheless, herbs are increasingly being taken seriously and studied for their effectiveness as medicines. The evidence is fairly impressive for some herbs. St. John's wort and ginkgo are probably the best studied, with double-blind trials that involved enough participants to really mean something.

Garlic too has a strong research record. More than 28 controlled clinical studies have been published in the last 20 years on the medicinal use of garlic for high blood cholesterol. Taken together, these studies strongly indicate that certain forms of garlic can reduce the level of total cholesterol in the blood. In the following sections, I'll describe the evidence in some detail. But first, I will discuss the nature of a properly designed scientific study.

How Do We Know a Treatment Really Works?

Determining whether a treatment is effective is not as simple as it might sound. It's not enough to show that the people who took the treatment improved. It also has to be shown that the improvement was actually *caused by* the treatment. For example, let's say that a doctor claims to have found the cure for the common cold. This doctor gives 20 individuals a dose of the new "cure," and voilá!—within 2 weeks, every person has completely recovered. But since most people with colds get better within 2 weeks anyway, this "study" gives us no evidence that the treatment had any effect at all.

Another problem for researchers is the well-known "placebo effect." Doctors have long noticed that people tend to get better whenever they take a treatment they believe might help them. Even treatment with placebo—a nonmedicinal substance such as a sugar pill—can make people feel better if they believe it is medicine. Also, when people believe they are taking an effective treatment, they may be more conscientious about taking other steps that can help them, such as improving their diet and increasing exercise. This can produce benefits even if the treatment itself is ineffective.

In order to get around this problem, scientists use what are called "double-blind placebo-controlled studies." The way such studies work is as follows: One group of study participants receives the real treatment (the treatment group), while the other group receives a fake treatment (the placebo control group). Neither group knows whether it's getting the real treatment or placebo (they are "blind").

Furthermore, the researchers administering placebo and real treatment are also kept in the dark about which group is receiving which treatment (making it a "double-blind" experiment). This last part is important, because it prevents the researchers from unintentionally tipping off the study participants, or unconsciously biasing their evaluation of the results. If participants and researchers know who is getting a treatment, the study is called an "open trial," and it is usually not very meaningful.

Finally, the more participants there are in a study and the longer the time period it covers, the more confidence we have in the results.

The Mader Study

One of the best and certainly the largest study on the effectiveness of garlic for high cholesterol was conducted in Germany, and the results were published in 1990.[5] Called the Mader study after its principal researcher, its results strongly suggest that regular use of garlic can lower cholesterol levels by an average of 12%. Although not perfect, the study was well designed, properly reported, and definitely worth taking seriously.

The Mader study results strongly suggest that regular use of garlic can lower cholesterol levels by an average of 12%.

This double-blind placebo-controlled trial enrolled 261 individuals selected from 30 different medical offices. Participants were randomly divided into two groups. One of the groups was given placebo. The other received four 200 mg garlic tablets each day. The garlic used in this study was a powder form standardized to contain 1.3% alliin. (See How to Take Garlic for more information on standardized herbal extracts.) At the beginning of the study, participants had total cholesterol levels that averaged about 265 mg/dL, significantly higher than what is considered healthy. Cholesterol levels were measured every month for 4 months.

The results as they developed over this time period were impressive. In the group that received garlic, there was a steady decline in total cholesterol with each blood sample, but there was little change in the placebo group. At the end of 4 months, cholesterol levels in the garlic group had fallen from an average of about 265 mg/dL to 235 mg/dL, a 12% improvement. By comparison, there was only a 3% improvement in the placebo group. Triglyceride levels also fell significantly—by 17% in the treated group, as compared to only 2% in the placebo group. (See figure 3.)

Whenever you see good results in a study like this, you have to ask one question: Were the results statistically significant?

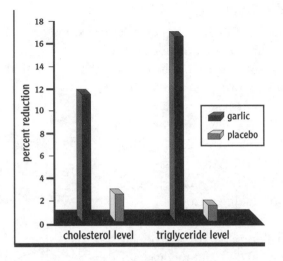

Figure 3. *Reduction in cholesterol and triglyceride levels after 4 months in a double-blind study* (Mader, 1990)

That is, do they really mean anything, or could they have happened by chance? If you flip a coin 20 times and it comes up heads 14 times, you can't really conclude from this that the coin is biased. But if you flip it 261 times and it comes up heads 200 times, you can be pretty sure something is going on.

Similarly, medical studies can be mathematically analyzed to determine whether their results are meaningful. There is more than one way to do this, and some methods have higher standards than others. In the case of this study, one of the strictest mathematical techniques was used (technically, the U-test for study power). The results showed that these outcomes were extremely unlikely to have happened by chance.

The Mader study wasn't perfect, however. One problem was rather difficult to get around: garlic's odor. Twenty-one percent of study participants taking garlic had either noticed the odor themselves or heard others commenting on it. This gave them the clue that they were receiving the treatment rather than the placebo. In a double-blind study, as we've seen, participants are not supposed to know whether they're receiving the treatment or placebo. If 21% of the treatment group knew what they were receiving, this reduces the validity of the study. But it's not quite as bad as it sounds. Reportedly, 9% of the placebo group also claimed to smell a garlic odor on their bodies, which means that many people taking the placebo believed they were getting the treatment. Also, keep in mind that in many double-blind studies of drugs, participants may be able to guess which group they are in based on the drug's side effects.[6] Studies are seldom perfect.

Perhaps the most unfortunate aspect of this study was that it failed to evaluate garlic's effects on HDL and LDL cholesterol, which are actually more important than total cholesterol. Still, even with its flaws, this study gives us solid evidence that garlic is an effective treatment for high cholesterol.

HDL and LDL

A study reported in 1993 did look at garlic's effects on HDL and LDL. It found positive results with LDL, but no significant change in HDL. This double-blind placebo-controlled study enrolled 42 people whose total cholesterol levels were above 220 mg/dL.[7] Those in the treatment group took 300 mg of garlic powder (standardized to 1.3% alliin content) 3 times a day; slightly more than in the Mader study. Researchers measured total cholesterol, LDL cholesterol, HDL cholesterol, triglycerides, glucose (blood sugar), blood pressure, and heart rate during the 12-week study.

At the end of 12 weeks, the treatment group's total cholesterol had fallen from an average 262 mg/dL to 247 mg/dL, a 6% reduction. LDL ("bad") cholesterol decreased from 188 mg/dL to 168 mg/dL, an impressive 11% decrease. However, there was no significant change in the treatment group's HDL ("good") cholesterol levels. In the placebo group, none of these measures changed significantly.

While not a large study, this trial does suggest that garlic can improve LDL levels. However, more research is clearly needed.

Meta-Analysis: Pooling Study Results

Besides the studies mentioned above, there have been at least two dozen other studies of garlic and its effects on cholesterol. In 1994, a group of researchers reviewed all the studies available up until that time.[8] Because some of the studies were less well-designed than others, they carefully evaluated all of them and settled on 16 that were acceptable. The other 9 were rejected for many reasons, mainly because the studies were too short or the information published in the original paper was missing important data.

The 16 accepted trials included a total of 952 participants. When all the data was pooled (using a special method called a *meta-analysis),* the results showed that garlic can reduce total cholesterol levels by an average of 10 to 12% over placebo, and can reduce triglycerides by 13%. There was not enough information in the studies to evaluate garlic's effects on HDL and LDL.

Even these 16 studies were not perfect. A different meta-analysis performed in 1993 was much more strict about which studies it would accept. Only 5 studies made it into the pool for review.[9] The total number of people enrolled in these 5 double-blind trials was 365. Pooling all the results, garlic appeared to lower cholesterol by about 9% more than placebo, slightly lower than in the other more generous meta-analysis, but still meaningful.

Aged Garlic May Be Effective

Nearly all the studies that have found garlic effective at reducing cholesterol used powdered garlic standardized to its alliin content. However, several studies used garlic that was simply aged, without any attempt to keep alliin intact. Because its processing is simpler, aged garlic is relatively inexpensive. There is some evidence that aged garlic may also lower cholesterol, but it may not lower it to the same extent as garlic processed to preserve the alliin.

In one study, 41 men with moderately high cholesterol took either placebo or 7.2 g of aged garlic extract daily for 4 to 6 months.[10] Aged garlic reduced total cholesterol by 6.1% more than placebo, and reduced LDL by 4.6% more than placebo.

While positive, these results were less impressive than what has been seen in studies of garlic powder standardized to 1.3% alliin. However, since there have not been any head-to-head comparisons, we can't really say for sure that aged garlic is less effective than standardized powdered garlic. Nonetheless, many experts suspect that it is weaker because it contains fewer of the probable active ingredients.

Garlic Oil: Not Effective

Garlic oil contains even fewer constituents of garlic than aged garlic, and it is not effective at reducing cholesterol.[11,12] This has been known for some time, but yet another study showing that it does not work was published in the *Journal of the American Medical Association* in 1998. The researchers performed a double-blind placebo-controlled crossover study of 25 individuals with moderately high cholesterol.[13] Participants were given either 5 mg of a commercial garlic oil (which is essentially garlic oil diluted in vegetable oil) or placebo for a period of 12 weeks. At the end of the study, there was no change in blood cholesterol.

Garlic oil contains even fewer constituents of garlic than aged garlic, and it is not effective at reducing cholesterol.

These results were no surprise. We already know that garlic oil doesn't work. Widespread media coverage misled much of the public by trying to use these results to "prove" that *all* forms of garlic are ineffective.

Negative Studies of Garlic Powder

One major study using standardized garlic powder did not come up with positive results. In 1996, the same researchers who performed the 1994 meta-analysis ran their own double-blind placebo-controlled trial, and to their own surprise came up with negative results.[14] The principal author expressed clear dismay at finding garlic ineffective, but nonetheless had the courage to publish the results.

In this study, a total of 115 individuals were followed for 6 months. Half received 900 mg of dried garlic powder daily (standardized to 1.3% allicin) and the other half received a matching placebo that was coated with garlic powder (too little to produce any therapeutic effect) so it would be indistinguishable from the actual garlic tablet. The results showed no benefits in any measured factors, including total cholesterol, triglycerides, LDL, or HDL levels.

What is the explanation for this discrepancy? One possibility, of course, is that garlic doesn't really work. But it is hard to ignore the sheer number of positive studies of garlic that came before it. Another possibility is that there was some feature of this study that would mask garlic's real effects. The likely suspect is diet. In this study, all participants were placed on a standard cholesterol-lowering diet. The researcher's purpose was to make sure that differences in individual dietary habits did not accidentally skew the results. However, since diet does have a significant effect on cholesterol levels, it is possible that very real benefits from garlic were covered over by the very real benefits of diet. In other words, maybe if you can manage to improve your diet, taking garlic doesn't provide any additional benefit. Perhaps garlic is most effective for people who, like many of us, find it very hard to make positive dietary changes.

Another study that found no benefits with garlic also made use of intentional dietary changes,[15] and a third was too small to mean much.[16] On balance, the evidence that garlic really works is very strong.

Garlic Versus Conventional Medications

To date, only one study has been published comparing the efficacy of garlic to that of a conventional drug in reducing cholesterol and triglycerides, and it must be taken with a grain of salt.

In 1992, a group of German researchers conducted a double-blind study comparing standardized garlic powder to bezafibrate (a cholesterol-lowering drug prescribed in Germany).[17] Ninety-eight participants were enrolled and randomly assigned to receive either garlic or bezafibrate. The results over 12 weeks showed that 900 mg of standardized garlic powder daily was equally effective to 600 mg of bezafibrate. Both reduced total cholesterol by about 25%.

This study has been widely quoted in the alternative press as proof that garlic is just as effective as drugs. But again all of the participants were put on a cholesterol-lowering diet during the study. Real differences between the two treatments may have been overridden by the powerful benefits of a healthy diet. One hint that this may be so is the remarkable extent of cholesterol reduction: 25% is higher than what would be expected with either garlic or bezafibrate alone.

Furthermore, bezafibrate is not as powerful as the most popular class of cholesterol-lowering drugs, the statins. As shown in chapter 6, the statin drugs regularly lower cholesterol by 25%. If you compare this with garlic's 10 to 12% as reported in most studies, it is clear that the medications are more powerful.

However, there is one way that garlic does seem to be preferable to drug treatment: risks and side effects. Garlic is associated with few side effects other than bad breath, and no significant risk of toxicity. This may be a significant advantage over drug treatments for people with mildly elevated cholesterol. See Safety Issues with Garlic for more information on garlic and its side effects.

How Does Garlic Work?

The exact mechanism by which garlic lowers cholesterol is not really clear, although we have some intriguing clues. While no one chemical in garlic has been shown to be the single active ingredient, most researchers would probably agree that the sulfur-containing compounds are responsible for the cholesterol-lowering effect.

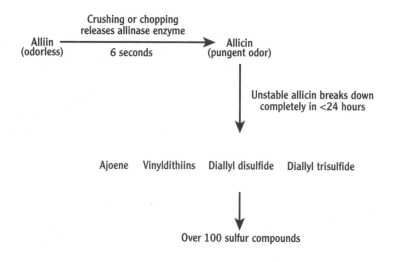

Figure 4. *Breakdown of garlic's sulfur-containing compounds*

Intact garlic contains an odorless chemical called alliin. Most of the studies described in this chapter used a form of garlic in which alliin is carefully preserved. Once in the body, the alliin breaks down into allicin and other substances including ajoene, vinyldithiins, diallyl disulfide, and diallyl trisulfide (see figure 4).These substances are rapidly absorbed.[18] These garlic constituents then help decrease the production of cholesterol.

In an animal study, garlic was found to inhibit an enzyme called HMG-CoA reductase.[19] The body uses this enzyme to manufacture cholesterol. The most widely used and effective class of cholesterol-lowering drugs, the statin drugs, also inhibits HMG-CoA reductase (see Safety Issues with Garlic). When this enzyme is inhibited, cholesterol levels fall.

What this study didn't examine carefully was the question of which constituents in garlic contributed to the positive effects. Two "test tube" studies on cells from rats have investigated this issue.[20,21] These studies found that allicin inhibits HMG-CoA reductase more profoundly than the other sulfur compounds, but substances such as diallyl disulfide and vinyldithiins are also effective. Garlic constituents also appear to inhibit another important cholesterol-producing enzyme as well—14-alpha demethylase. Many other studies have examined the effects of various garlic constituents.[22–25]

The upshot of all these studies appears to be that garlic produces its effects on cholesterol in more than one way, and its various constituents may work together to produce a combined effect. However, there is still much we do not know.

Beyond Cholesterol: Garlic's Other Potential Benefits for Your Arteries

As the studies discussed in The Scientific Evidence show, garlic appears to significantly lower total cholesterol levels. But garlic may offer other benefits for treating and preventing atherosclerosis. Several double-blind studies suggest that garlic modestly, but meaningfully, reduces blood pressure, which is a known risk factor for atherosclerosis. The combined benefits of reducing both cholesterol and blood pressure make garlic a promising all-around preventive treatment for atherosclerosis. Not only that, one ground-breaking study suggests that garlic's usefulness in treating and preventing atherosclerosis goes beyond its effects on either cholesterol or blood pressure. So we have to look further. Some possibilities for other positive effects include garlic's known ability to "thin" the blood and fight free radicals.

This chapter explores all the other ways garlic may protect your arteries. It also presents evidence from an exciting study, which suggests that regular use of garlic can reduce the risk of a heart attack.

Several double-blind studies suggest that garlic modestly, but meaningfully, reduces blood pressure, which is a known risk factor for atherosclerosis.

Garlic and High Blood Pressure

There is considerable evidence that garlic can reduce high blood pressure (or *hypertension*), at least modestly. Some of this evidence comes from animal studies.[26,27] Additionally, in studies evaluating garlic's effects on cholesterol, researchers have noticed reductions in blood pressure as a kind of positive "side effect." Finally, a few human studies have focused directly on garlic's effect on blood pressure as their primary interest. The overall results suggest that garlic can indeed meaningfully reduce blood pressure.

One of the best studies of garlic's effects on high blood pressure was a 1990 double-blind placebo-controlled study of 47 individuals.[28] This 12-week trial enrolled people with mild hypertension, with average blood pressure readings of about 170/100 mm Hg (millimeters of mercury—normal is 140/90 or lower). Participants were given either 600 mg of garlic powder or a similar-looking placebo.

At the end of the study, the group given garlic showed a significant reduction in blood pressure compared to the placebo group. The diastolic blood pressure (the bottom number in blood pressure readings) had fallen by about 13 mm Hg, whereas those taking placebo had no significant change.

Systolic blood pressure (the top number of the blood pressure reading) also fell considerably in the group taking the garlic. There was a 19 mm Hg average drop in the garlic group versus no significant change in the placebo group.

In other words, participants who began with a reading of 170/100 ended up with a much closer to normal blood pressure of 151/89. (See figures 5 and 6.) Although the systolic blood pressure reading was still too high, overall, blood pressure was much better. There were no reports of side effects, and only three participants mentioned that they noticed a slight garlic odor.

Good results have been seen in many other studies as well. In 1994, Professor Christopher Silagy and Dr. Andrew Neil from Oxford University conducted a review of all the human studies published at that time on garlic's influence on blood

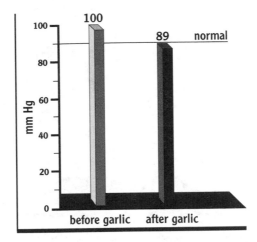

Figure 5. *Reduction in systolic blood pressure in treatment (garlic) group after 12 weeks in a double-blind study* (Auer, 1990)

pressure.[29] To be included in their review, each study had to use a double-blind design, last at least 4 weeks, and satisfy other requirements to ensure that the results were meaningful. Eight trials met these requirements. They all used dried garlic powder standardized to 1.3% alliin in doses ranging from 600 to 900 mg per day. The average duration of the trials was about 12 weeks, and a total of 415 subjects were involved. However, only three of the studies involved people with high blood pressure.

When pooled together, the overall results of these studies suggest that garlic can reduce blood pressure better than placebo, although the exact amount of the reduction varies from study to study. Improvements were similar to those seen in the 1990 study described above.

The authors of this meta-analysis caution that even the eight studies they accepted into the review were not top-notch; they all suffered from a number of technical flaws. We really need larger, longer, and better designed studies. Nonetheless, the available evidence does suggest that garlic can meaningfully reduce blood pressure. The researchers point out that this effect, if sustained over a long period of time, could add up to a

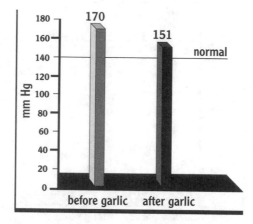

Figure 6. *Reduction in diastolic blood pressure in treatment (garlic) group after 12 weeks in a double-blind study* (Auer, 1990)

major health benefit, reducing strokes by 30 to 40% and heart disease by 20 to 25%.

How Does Garlic Work to Lower High Blood Pressure?

Although there are several theories that try to explain how garlic might work to reduce blood pressure, we don't really know for sure which one is correct. Our best guess is that garlic dilates blood vessels. When the vessels become wider, more blood can flow through with less resistance, reducing blood pressure.

But how does garlic dilate blood vessels? One theory suggests that garlic relaxes the artery walls by stimulating the production of nitric oxide.[30,31] Nitric oxide is a natural substance that the body itself releases to relax the muscles that line arteries. However, this theory is far from proven.[32]

Another theory suggests that garlic may work like a family of blood pressure medications known as "calcium channel blockers." These drugs relax the artery wall by blocking the entrance of calcium into cells, thereby causing them to relax (for reasons that are too complex to delve into here). Several laboratory studies have found that both garlic and its individual constituents can affect the way calcium moves into smooth muscle cells.[33,34] However, as yet, there have been no human studies showing the same effect.

The bottom line is that while garlic does appear to reduce blood pressure, we don't know exactly how it works.

Cholesterol and Blood Pressure Aren't the Whole Story

Given that garlic can reduce cholesterol and blood pressure, one would certainly expect it to reduce the rate of atherosclerosis. Animal studies definitely indicate that this is the case. According to a review published in 1997, at least 16 controlled animal studies have been performed evaluating garlic's effects on atherosclerosis.[35] Twelve of the studies found that garlic protects against the formation of atherosclerosis. Furthermore, three studies found that it can actually reverse atherosclerosis. Only one study did not find any benefit.

While these results are exciting, you have to keep in mind that there was a certain artificiality to all of them. These were not laboratory animals that just happened to develop atherosclerosis; rather, researchers stimulated it by one artificial means or another. In some studies, an artery wall was deliberately damaged, while in others, animals were fed a diet designed to dramatically speed atherosclerosis. Still, these findings are definitely promising, and they deserve to be taken seriously.

Garlic might work to reduce blood pressure by dilating blood vessels. When the vessels become wider, more blood can flow through with less resistance, reducing blood pressure.

It's much harder to study atherosclerosis in people. Not only would it be unethical to deliberately give people atherosclerosis, most methods used to measure the extent of mild atherosclerosis are dangerous or at least unpleasant.

However, a recent study used a very clever approach to discover whether garlic reduces atherosclerosis in people. This study, published in 1997, estimated the extent of atherosclerosis by looking at the elasticity of the largest artery in the body, the aorta.[36] As atherosclerosis advances, the aorta becomes stiffer. In general, the older you are, the stiffer the aorta becomes, because just about everyone develops some atherosclerosis over time. There is a special (and extremely technical) technique known as *pulse wave velocity measurement* that can evaluate the elasticity of the aorta without posing any risk to the participant.

The study followed 101 matched pairs of people between ages 50 and 80, who were carefully selected to be similar in every important way except for their use of garlic. One group consisted of those who reported taking more than 300 mg of standardized garlic powder per day for at least 2 years. The other group was similar in age, sex, and weight but did not take garlic on a regular basis.

Garlic's "blood-thinning" effects may be the explanation for its ability to treat and prevent atherosclerosis.

These two groups were then evaluated using the pulse wave velocity measurement technique. The results were positive and unmistakable: Individuals who used garlic regularly had much more flexible aortas. Thus, regular garlic use was associated with less atherosclerosis. This strongly suggests that garlic use can slow down the development of atherosclerosis. (It is always possible in studies of this type that other factors were involved, and the use of garlic was only a coincidence. However, this isn't likely.)

This study had one surprising feature: People taking garlic developed less atherosclerosis even though their cholesterol level and blood pressure were identical (on average) to those who did not take it. This suggests that garlic's atherosclerosis-

---

Can Garlic's "Blood-Thinning" Effects Be Dangerous?

One patient read that garlic decreased blood clotting, and she became concerned that she might bleed to death if she cut herself. Garlic is definitely not this powerful! However, garlic's influence on blood clotting does suggest that it might be risky to combine it with blood-thinning drugs, or perhaps even natural supplements that also thin the blood. It also might not be a good idea to take garlic immediately before or after surgery or labor and delivery, and people with blood clotting disorders should definitely seek medical advice. For more information, see Safety Issues with Garlic.

---

fighting powers are greater than the sum of its effects on cholesterol and blood pressure. Some other action or actions must be at work as well.

Garlic and Blood Clotting (Hemostasis)

Garlic's "blood-thinning" effects may be the explanation for its ability to treat and prevent atherosclerosis. Garlic appears to both help prevent blood clots from forming, and help break down clots that have already developed. (For a refresher, go to chapter 1 for information on how blood clots play a role in atherosclerosis.) These clots not only add to the layer of plaque coating blood vessel walls; they can also break loose and become lodged further down the bloodstream, causing a stroke or heart attack.

One commonly prescribed preventive treatment for heart disease is taking one baby aspirin a day. Aspirin is a blood thinner, which is believed to be at least one reason why it helps. It works by interfering with platelets, cells that start the formation of a clot. Platelets (see chapter 1) normally circulate throughout our arteries and veins, waiting to repair any leaks. When they find an injured or leaking artery, they attach to it, quickly forming a plug.

Unfortunately, platelets see atherosclerosis as "injury" to our bodies, and act as if the plaque was a bleeding artery. The platelets surround the plaque and begin to stick to both the lesion and each other. This sets off a cascade of events which, as we've seen, can lead to a disaster for your health. Chemicals released by platelets may also accelerate atherosclerosis.

Like aspirin, one of the ways garlic intervenes in clot formation is by keeping the platelets from sticking to each other. If the platelets can't clump easily, then a clot is less likely to form. Several studies have found that garlic and its constituents can reduce the ability of platelets to adhere to each other and to plaque.[37–41]

Warning: If you have been advised to take aspirin to help prevent heart attacks, I do not recommend substituting garlic for it except on the advice of a physician. We don't know if garlic is as effective as aspirin for this purpose.

Garlic has another effect besides helping prevent clots from forming. It seems to help break down existing blood clots. It does so by dissolving a protein called *fibrin,* which is the "webbing" of a clot.[42,43] This dissolving action is called *fibrinolysis.* Clot-dissolving drugs are used in the immediate stages after a heart attack or stroke.

The drugs used to break down clots immediately after heart attacks are much more potent—too potent to be taken long term. Garlic's effect certainly doesn't seem to be strong enough to make garlic a good alternative to drugs in emergencies. But perhaps garlic will prove to be effective enough to be used as a preventive measure in treating blood clots. At this point, we don't have the answer. Interestingly, even cooked garlic seems to dissolve clots to some extent.[44]

Garlic As an Antioxidant

One theory suggests that free radicals are an important cause of atherosclerosis (see chapter 1). Free radicals are naturally occurring molecules that can damage many of our tissues. They can also attack LDL ("bad") cholesterol and make it even more harmful to arteries.

A number of substances called *antioxidants* help the body combat the damaging effects of oxidation. For example, vitamin E is a potent antioxidant that has been found to reduce the incidence of heart disease. (For more information on vitamin E, see chapter 3, as well as *The Natural Pharmacist: Heart Disease Prevention.*)

Garlic, too, is a potent antioxidant, and it appears to protect LDL cholesterol from free radicals.[45–48] Several studies have identified some of garlic's sulfur compounds as antioxidants, including alliin and allicin as well as two other compounds called S-allyl cysteine and diallyl disulfide.[49,50] Other studies on garlic indicate that it is also an effective neutralizer of free radicals.[51,52]

> **Garlic appears to both help prevent blood clots from forming, and help break down clots that have already developed.**

Does Garlic Reduce Deaths from Heart Disease?

Although all the findings described in this chapter are intriguing, the bottom-line question is whether the regular use of garlic actually prevents death due to heart disease. There is evidence showing that various cholesterol-lowering medications may provide this important benefit (see chapter 6). There is also some evidence in favor of aspirin and vitamin E.

A controlled study published in 1989 provides evidence that garlic, too, may prevent heart attacks and heart attack death. This 3-year study followed 432 individuals who had previously suffered a heart attack.[53] Half of the participants received fresh squeezed garlic juice in milk (yum!) equivalent to about 2 g daily of fresh garlic, while the others did not receive any treatment. All participants continued to take whatever standard medications they had been prescribed. The results were

very impressive. Those who had taken the garlic had a significant reduction in both mortality from heart attacks (45%) and
in the recurrence of heart attacks (35%). This finding is significant because it suggests that garlic's effects are not just theoretically beneficial, but that they actually add up to longer life and
fewer heart attacks. After all, it is perfectly possible that a treatment that improves some risk factors for heart disease might
produce other hidden negative effects as well, producing an
overall negative outcome in certain cases. It is reassuring to see
some evidence suggesting that, all things considered, garlic produced a strong net benefit.

However, there was a severe problem with this study: It
wasn't blinded (see How Do We Know a Treatment Really
Works? for a discussion of double-blind studies). Because the
participants knew whether they were receiving garlic or not,
there was room for the power of suggestion to play its usual
confusing role. Can the power of suggestion protect a person
from heart attacks? It's possible. If the study had been blinded,
we could be more confident of its results. As it is, we'll have to
wait for further research to add to our bottom-line knowledge
of garlic's power against heart disease.

How to Take Garlic

As you will see, knowing exactly which type of garlic to take and
how much to take is a bit more complicated than it sounds. Finding the proper dosage of herbs and comparing different products
involves numerous issues that simply don't exist with drugs.

A good place to start is to follow the recommendations of
Germany's Commission E. This official governmental agency
performs a job similar to that of the U.S. Food and Drug Administration (FDA), only it is specifically focused on herbs (see Garlic and Modern Medicine). Commission E suggests the following
daily dose of garlic for the purpose of lowering cholesterol and
preventing atherosclerosis: 4 grams of fresh raw garlic (roughly 1
very large clove or 2 average-sized ones) or the equivalent daily.

Because most people don't like raw garlic, garlic powder preparations are usually used instead. The best-studied form is a preparation of garlic standardized to contain 1.3% alliin. The proper dose of this type of garlic is 300 mg taken 2 to 3 times daily. The label may say, "provides 10 mg (or 10,000 mcg) alliin daily" or "provides 4 mg (4000 mcg) allicin potential daily."

This chapter will help you understand what form of garlic is best to take. It will also fill you in on what to expect when you take garlic and when you should not rely on this herb.

What Is a Standardized Herbal Extract?

Many forms of garlic appear on supermarket shelves, and some of them claim to be superior to the other products. However, there is no foolproof way to decide which one is best. We still aren't absolutely sure which of garlic's ingredients are the most important. For this reason, it is very difficult to compare products reliably.

A standardized herbal extract is a concentrated form of an herb, processed to contain a fixed percentage of one or more of its ingredients.

Virtually all popular herbal treatments present this quandary. In this sense at least, herbs are fundamentally different from pharmaceuticals. When you purchase a drug, you know exactly what you are getting and how much. Drugs are single chemicals that can be measured and quantified down to their molecular structure. Thus, a tablet of Extra Strength Tylenol contains 500 mg of acetaminophen, no matter where or when you buy it. If you wish to buy generic acetaminophen, you can simply read the label and see how much each tablet contains.

But with herbal medicine, you can't be sure that two different batches of the same herb have the same potency. Herbs aren't interchangeable like drugs. An herb is a living organism that contains hundreds or thousands of chemicals in varying quantities. The soil the herb grew in, the weather, the plants that flourished around it, and the conditions under which it was harvested and stored—all of these factors will influence the chemical makeup of what you see on the shelf. Genetics can also have an influence. Different strains of garlic undoubtedly have different proportions of certain chemicals.

This complication is precisely why medical scientists made drugs out of herbs in the first place. They wanted something reliable, reproducible, and trustworthy year to year and batch to batch. A traditional herbalist might roughly evaluate the potency of a given herb by looking at it closely, touching it, and smelling it. However, this isn't very scientific. In the modern world, treatments need to be manufactured in a more objective manner.

To partially overcome this problem, modern herbalists often use what is known as a *standardized herbal extract.* This is a concentrated form of an herb, processed to contain a fixed percentage of one or more ingredients. Thus, the ultimate product is said to be standardized to that ingredient.

In the case of garlic, most manufacturers standardize to alliin content. For example, many clinical studies of garlic (see The Scientific Evidence and Beyond Cholesterol: Garlic's Other Potential Benefits for Your Arteries) employed an extract standardized to contain 1.3% alliin. Alliin has been selected as the standardizing ingredient because of evidence that it—and the allicin it breaks down into—are the active ingredients in garlic.

When you use a standardized extract, you have some reason to believe that one garlic pill is similar in strength to the others. The big advantage of this method is that it allows herbs to be studied in the same kind of rigorous trials as drugs; a necessity if we wish to know for sure whether a traditional herbal treatment really works.

Keep in mind that standardization isn't foolproof. A standardized herbal extract capsule is rated only according to its level of one—or at most, a few—ingredients. Hundreds or thousands of other ingredients may still vary widely from pill to pill. They may vary even more from manufacturer to manufac-

Table 1. Clinical Human Studies on Garlic

Form of Garlic	Average Dose Used	Number of Studies	Cholesterol-Lowering Effect
Dried garlic powder	600–900 mg	28	10–25%
Aged garlic	1–7.2 g	6	7–10%
Fresh garlic	1–2 cloves	4	10%
Garlic oil	4–18 mg	6	No benefit

turer, based on differences in production method, even when the end result has a fixed amount of alliin.

This wouldn't matter if we were sure that alliin was the only active ingredient. In fact, if we knew it were, we could just extract alliin and use it as a drug. However, garlic's effects are probably due to many compounds, which may be effective singly or only in combination. In one study (see Aged Garlic May Be Effective), aged garlic lowered cholesterol, and aged garlic has little to no alliin in it at all. It does contain many other sulfur-based substances. Fried garlic also contains little alliin, but it can affect blood clotting (see Garlic and Blood Clotting (Hemostasis)). Two products with identical alliin content may differ in other ingredients, and therefore in overall effectiveness. We don't know how to determine in advance just how effective a particular garlic formulation really is. There's still one more problem with garlic: Its ingredients are unstable and easily break down into other compounds. Even if a product contains certain ingredients when it's manufactured, the product on the shelf that you ultimately purchase may have spontaneously changed so much that its constituents are quite different.

Given all that we don't know, it is perfectly possible that an unstandardized product may be just as effective as a standardized one. Still, keep in mind that garlic powder standardized to alliin content has been the predominant form used in double-blind trials. So, for now, it is probably the most reliable choice.

Table 1 gives a breakdown of the forms of garlic used in studies. Garlic powder has been used in about 65% of studies, garlic oil in 13% of studies, aged garlic in 12%, and fresh garlic in 10%. All of them have been found effective, except garlic oil.

One day, perhaps, we'll know precisely which ingredients in garlic are important for reducing cholesterol and atherosclerosis, and we'll be able to precisely standardize garlic products. But for now, there's a bit of trial and error involved.

Garlic has one advantage over many other herbs: It's a widely available food. If you don't find any effect with garlic powder or an aged garlic product, you can always try whole garlic for a while to see whether the problem was the garlic itself or just the preparation. And, as an added benefit, if you like its taste, whole garlic can be delicious as well as good for you.

Garlic Preparations

Companies that make herbs produce many different forms of garlic. Some products boast that they are "odorless" or "odor free," while others claim that odor is a sign of a high-quality product. In the following section, I hope to clarify how these products are made, so you can make an informed decision about which one is best for you.

Powdered Garlic

It is well accepted that alliin and allicin break down rapidly soon after fresh garlic is cut or crushed. But in order to be made into a powder capable of fitting into a capsule or tablet, garlic has to be crushed. Manufacturers have puzzled over the problem of keeping these substances intact in their garlic products, and have come up with some ingenious solutions.

One method is to destroy the enzyme allinase. Allinase is what converts alliin into allicin (see chapter 1 and The Scientific Evidence later in this chapter). Allicin then breaks down into other substances. By first eliminating allinase, manufacturers can then crush, dry, and powder the garlic to their hearts' content. This powder contains fairly high levels of alliin, but no allicin, because there is no allinase to make it.

After the drying process is completed, allinase is added back to the dried powder, which is made into hard capsules. When dry, allinase cannot do its work. This capsule will therefore remain stable until it comes into contact with the fluids in the intestines. At that point, the allinase is activated, and starts turning alliin to allicin.

> In the case of garlic, many manufacturers standardize to alliin because of the evidence that it may be an active ingredient.

One of the advantages of this form of garlic is that it contains alliin in its original form. It is a relatively simple matter to standardize such products to alliin content. Another benefit is that it is relatively odorless, because there is no allicin in the product until it reaches your intestines. Allicin is mostly responsible for garlic's strong odor (see What Is in Garlic?). Therefore, some people find this form of garlic more desirable. (There is still some smell on your breath and through the pores of your skin from the allicin that's formed inside your body.)

Another method that works equally well involves slicing the garlic into thin pieces, then rapidly drying it. Allicin is formed along the borders of each slice, but inside the dried slice, alliin and allinase don't interact. The pieces can then be safely ground into a powder without triggering the reaction. Again, the sliced garlic powder becomes activated when it comes into contact with the moisture of the intestines, releasing allicin.

This method of drying garlic maintains the sulfur compounds, such as alliin and sulfides, originally found in fresh garlic. However, because some allicin was activated on the face of each slice, this kind of garlic has a slightly garlicky odor.

Like the other powdered capsules mentioned above, the advantage of this kind of product is that it can be standardized to alliin content. Most of the controlled clinical studies on garlic have used this form.

However, with both of these types of powdered garlic preparations, we have the problem of not knowing exactly how much allicin gets produced in the intestines. Such products may state a certain "allicin potential" or "allicin yield," referring to the amount of allicin the manufacturer believes will be released in the intestines, but this is hard to determine precisely, and may be more wishful thinking than anything else.

To get around this, some manufacturers crush the garlic and allow allicin to form, and then artificially stabilize it. Since such products do have an odor, they are usually made into coated tablets that open up somewhere in the intestines. When the tablet reaches the intestines, the allicin is released.

This product is good because it lets us quantify the amount of allicin precisely. It can be standardized to actual allicin content instead of a hypothetical allicin yield. However, this form of garlic is definitely not odor free, and those who don't like the smell of garlic may find it unpleasant. Another problem is that if the allicin is too well stabilized, it may not break down into other compounds the way it does with other forms of garlic. Some of allicin's breakdown products may play an important role in reducing cholesterol or heart disease. Also, when alliin is converted into allicin, it produces several other compounds. Some of these might be important, but we don't know if they survive this processing method.

So which type of powdered garlic should you get? I recommend matching the form used in the studies as closely as possible. Purchase a brand that states its alliin content.

Aged Garlic

Have you heard of the old French traditional medicine, Four Thieves Vinegar (see What Was Garlic Used for Historically?)? It was originally made from garlic steeped in wine or vinegar. In a sense, it was the earliest use of an aged garlic product for medicinal purposes. Modern day aged garlic preparations are primarily produced by a technique developed in Japan.

The process of making aged garlic involves chopping or slicing garlic and placing it in alcohol for up to 2 years. The tanks that hold the garlic mixture are kept cool to avoid any decomposition of the garlic compounds by heat. This long aging process allows the many oil-soluble, sulfur-containing compounds, such as alliin, allicin, sulfides, and vinyldithiins, to be broken down into more stable by-products. Part of the reason some scientists prefer this form of garlic is precisely because it *doesn't* contain any allicin. Some Japanese researchers have argued that allicin is harmful, and that aged garlic is safer. While other authorities do not agree, most of the safety studies done on the subject (see Safety Issues with Garlic) have used aged garlic, and it is probably the one form that we know for sure is completely safe.

Modern day aged garlic preparations are primarily produced by a technique developed in Japan.

Nonetheless, the use of aged garlic remains controversial. Because it lacks alliin, allicin, and other constituents that are believed to be medically active in reducing cholesterol and heart disease, many authorities feel that it is distinctly inferior.

In fact, Germany's Commission E does not allow aged garlic to be sold as a cholesterol-lowering supplement. The Commission E specifies that anticholesterol garlic products must be equivalent to fresh, raw garlic, a requirement not met by aged garlic. Nevertheless, several studies suggest that aged garlic does work.[54–56]

Many people prefer aged garlic because it is truly odor-free, and it is very easy on the stomach. Because of its chemical composition, it may be the most tolerable form for people who are highly sensitive to garlic.

Options for Enjoying Fresh Garlic

If you decide to try fresh, whole garlic, there are some delicious alternatives to simply chewing up one clove at a time. Try eating it on your salad in a freshly made garlic dressing: Crush 1 or more cloves of garlic (a garlic press is a handy tool) and add olive oil and balsamic vinegar to taste. Experiment with different vinegars and seasonings such as oregano, basil, pepper, and mustard. (Keep in mind that if you put this dressing in the refrigerator, you are making aged garlic.)

If you like Middle Eastern food, you can make hummus: Blend some cooked, cooled garbanzo beans together and add small amounts, to taste, of tahini (sesame paste), olive oil, lemon juice, salt (if your blood pressure allows), and fresh garlic. Use it as a dip for vegetables, or spread it on pita bread.

Fresh Garlic

Fresh, raw garlic may be the strongest form of garlic available (at least theoretically). By definition, it contains all of the therapeutic ingredients present in garlic cloves. These ingredients are released during chewing. While this is certainly a cheap, easy way to take garlic, it has some serious problems—primarily the taste and smell.

Unless you live in a community where everyone eats a lot of garlic, you may find your neighbors standing at a considerable distance from you. Furthermore, fresh garlic can be quite painful in the mouth when you try to eat it. It may also irritate the intestines, causing heartburn and gas. (See Safety Issues with Garlic for a more thorough discussion of garlic's side effects.) For all these reasons, many people find it easier to take a pill rather than to eat a fresh clove every day.

However, if you're not sensitive to raw garlic and you don't mind the odor (which varies from one person to the next), it may be the best form overall. After all, the reason most of us

Hard-core garlic lovers will eat it raw in just about anything: pizza (sprinkle chopped, fresh garlic on a cooked pizza the minute it leaves the oven), soups and stews (use a garlic press to add fresh garlic just before serving), or even blended up in a vegetable-juice smoothie.

Of course, cooked garlic is found in many foods. Unfortunately, we don't know how effective it might be. We do know that it does not contain the same amount of active ingredients as freshly cut, raw garlic, so baking, roasting, sautéing, or frying your medicinal garlic may not give you the same cholesterol-lowering benefit. Regardless, eating plenty of cooked garlic probably can't hurt!

---

turn to herbs is that we want to use "natural" methods. The most natural (and least expensive) form of garlic is clearly garlic itself. As mentioned earlier in table 1, 4 studies have investigated fresh garlic and found results comparable to what has been seen with standardized powdered garlic.

Garlic Oil

Dating back to the 1920s, garlic oil was the original commercial garlic product made. It was first developed in Europe, and it is still widely used there. There are several methods for extracting garlic in oil, but none of them retain alliin or allicin.[57] Garlic oil products do, however, contain other important substances such as ajoene and vinyldithiins.

When oil is extracted from raw garlic, it is extremely concentrated. To counter the odor and potential stomach irritation it can cause, most manufacturers dilute it in a vegetable oil (such as soybean oil). Some commercial products may be diluted up to 100 times, meaning that 1 garlic oil capsule will only contain

1 drop of essential oil. As a result, you would have to take as many as 10 capsules to equal 1 small clove of garlic (and you still wouldn't be getting any alliin or allicin).

Garlic oil does not appear to reduce cholesterol levels. However, because it does seem to decrease the tendency toward blood clotting, it may still have beneficial effects in treating or preventing atherosclerosis. Nonetheless, due to the limited usefulness and lack of research on garlic oil, I recommend using other forms.

So Which Form Should You Buy?

Garlic powder standardized to 1.3% alliin content is probably your best bet, because it most closely resembles the form used in the majority of studies. Remember, your daily dose should supply 10,000 mcg (10 mg) of alliin, or 4,000 mcg (4 mg) of allicin potential. However, make sure to read the label carefully. Some forms of garlic will list alliin or allicin content "at the time of production," which of course tells you nothing about the amount of alliin or allicin it may still contain. A good product should state the amount of the garlic components at the time of *purchase*, not production!

> When you're looking in the store for a garlic product, read the label carefully. A good product should state the amount of the garlic components at the time of purchase, not production.

Aged garlic extract may be useful, but it doesn't contain alliin or allicin and is not standardized. Most of the successful studies on aged garlic have used 1 g daily, so you might want to start with this dose. If you aren't seeing results after a couple of months, increase the dose by 1 g at a time until your cholesterol starts to drop. As shown in the table 1, the clinical studies on aged garlic have used anywhere from 1 to 7.2 g daily. If you reach a daily dosage of 7.2 g and are not seeing results, consult your doctor to explore other options.

Other forms of garlic, such as tinctures (alcohol extracts) and garlic vinegar, are commonly sold in health-food stores. These types of garlic have a long historical use and may have some benefits. The problem is that the garlic content will vary tremendously, depending on how much garlic was used to make the preparation, how long the garlic was soaked in the fluid, and the type of fluid used. With so many unanswered questions about this preparation, it may be better for you to stick to a standardized product.

What to Expect When You Take Garlic

Like high blood pressure, high cholesterol is a silent disease. If you have mild to moderately elevated cholesterol, you probably had no idea it was high until your doctor tested your blood.

For this reason, you're not likely to *feel* your cholesterol or triglyceride levels decreasing. Additionally, once you start trying to lower your cholesterol, improvement will take awhile. Be patient, and remember that garlic works slowly. Wait 2 to 3 months before getting your cholesterol rechecked, and then see how you're doing. Like any other herb, garlic needs to be taken consistently for the benefits to appear. Taking a pill every now and then or eating garlic once a week is not likely to produce any results. Persistence is the key here.

Like any other medication or herb, garlic needs to be taken consistently for the benefits to appear. Persistence is the key.

Temporary Setbacks

A few studies suggest that garlic may produce a paradoxical and *temporary* elevation of cholesterol. For example, a double-blind placebo-controlled study in 1987 looked at the effects of aged garlic on blood lipids.[58]

To the researcher's dismay, the blood samples from the garlic group taken in the first 2 months showed an *increase* in total cholesterol and triglycerides. The researchers were ready to abandon the study right then, but luckily they came across a 1981 study that found the same phenomenon, except that the increase was only temporary and was followed by a longer-term decrease.[59] Sure enough, after the third month on garlic, the participants' total cholesterol and triglycerides, as well as their LDL ("bad") cholesterol levels, had gone down. In addition, their HDL ("good") cholesterol levels had gone up. At the end of 6 months, 65% of the participants on garlic had achieved healthy blood cholesterol and triglyceride levels. We're not sure why this brief increase in cholesterol and triglyceride levels occurs, but it has been observed in two other studies as well. One theory is that garlic causes cholesterol and triglycerides to shift out of the tissues and into the bloodstream. If you get your cholesterol measured during this phase, the test will show an increase. Eventually, cholesterol levels will fall as garlic gets down to its work of decreasing cholesterol production.

While this theory may be true, it has not been thoroughly researched. Also, this temporary rise doesn't always occur. Several studies have not found it, and many practitioners have never seen it in their patients. Then again, they may not have been doing monthly blood draws on their patients after starting them on garlic, because they expect garlic to take a few months to work. These practitioners usually have patients return after a few months for their first follow-up. It is possible that this effect happens from time to time, but it isn't caught because the blood isn't being retested soon enough. But if you are impatient and have your blood tested 1 month after getting started on garlic, you may see this happen. Don't be frightened. Your cholesterol and triglyceride levels should go down after about 3 months.

A Surprising "Side Effect"

Finally, although you should not *feel* any real changes when taking garlic, at least two studies suggest otherwise. Surprisingly, garlic powder improved mood and overall feelings of well-being, almost as if it were an antidepressant. This phenomenon has not been well researched, but it has been observed, and maybe you will experience it, too.

Surprisingly, garlic powder has been found to improve mood and overall feelings of well-being.

In one double-blind study, researchers used a test called EWL-60-S that provides a choice of 60 words the individuals can use to express their feelings in certain categories.[60] The results were surprising: In individuals given garlic, the scores showed that positive characteristics such as mood, concentration, and self-assurance went up, while negative characteristics like fatigue, irritability, and anxiety went down. There was no significant change in the placebo group.

What is going on here? Is garlic an antidepressant? This has never been claimed about garlic, but clearly more research should be done on this pleasant "side effect."

When Not to Take Garlic

Garlic isn't right for everybody. For example, if you have a fasting total cholesterol higher than 300 mg/dL despite a healthy lifestyle, garlic alone most definitely won't be strong enough to bring your cholesterol down to safe levels. You will almost surely need to take cholesterol-lowering drugs, preferably those in the statin family (see The Statin Family: Powerful Medications with Few Side Effects in chapter 6).

If your cholesterol is in the 250 to 300 mg/dL range, garlic and some of the other supplements described in chapters 3 and

4 might be able to bring it down to normal levels, especially if you also improve your lifestyle.

However, if despite all your best efforts, your cholesterol levels still remain too high, don't stubbornly insist on natural treatments. Heart disease and strokes are so serious that their risks may far outweigh the potential risks of using drugs. Please discuss this subject with your physician to obtain the most personalized information.

> **If despite all your best efforts, your cholesterol levels remain too high, don't stubbornly insist on natural treatments.**

Another situation in which garlic is not appropriate is if you are truly allergic to it. Although rare, a true garlic allergy is not the same thing as an intolerance or sensitivity that leads to minor symptoms such as gastrointestinal discomfort. An allergy is a physical reaction. In milder forms, it can manifest as a skin rash or other non-serious symptom, but in its more serious form, it can lead to a powerful reaction called *anaphylaxis*, which involves the entire body and can be dangerous. If you know that you are allergic to garlic, you should not take it.

Fortunately, allergic reactions to garlic are extremely uncommon. According to studies, it appears that only about 1% of those taking garlic have an allergic reaction to it, and most of these are minor. I have not seen any reports in the literature linking garlic to anaphylaxis, so this risk may be more theoretical than real. However, if you experience any of the following symptoms while taking garlic, discontinue it immediately and consult your physician: difficulty breathing, fever, redness of the skin, chest tightness, or loss of consciousness.

The following important safety issues are discussed further in Safety Issues with Garlic. First, because of its blood-thinning effects, garlic should probably not be combined with certain anticoagulant drugs, such as Coumadin (warfarin) or heparin. There may even be reason for concern if you are taking blood-thinning natural products, such as ginkgo, vitamin E, or feverfew. Also, you shouldn't take garlic if you are about to undergo—or have just undergone—surgery or labor and delivery. Also, those with certain diseases, such as pemphigus (a rare autoimmune disease that involves the skin and mucous membranes) or diabetes that is difficult to control, should also avoid garlic except under a doctor's supervision. Finally, because garlic thins the blood, people with any reason to worry about excessive bleeding need to use caution (see Safety Issues with Garlic for more details).

Treat the Whole Person

Simply taking a garlic pill isn't always going to solve your problems with high cholesterol. One of the principles of medicine given by Hippocrates, the father of medicine, is to "treat the whole person." This means that you should manage your high cholesterol as well as deal with the factors in your life that may have led to its becoming elevated in the first place.

Diet and exercise are definitely recommended as the first place to make changes before you undergo any other treatment.

Improving diet and increasing exercise are definitely recommended as the first steps to take before you undergo any more specific treatment. Admittedly, these can be the most challenging parts of your life to change. Our eating and behavioral patterns are deeply ingrained habits that often go back to childhood (see chapter 5).

Remember: Don't be discouraged if change seems slow to you. Just keep in mind that progress, even in small amounts, means you're still heading in the right direction.

Safety Issues with Garlic

When garlic is taken at the recommended doses, it appears to be a safe therapy. In fact, the U.S. Food and Drug Administration (FDA) classifies garlic on its GRAS list, an acronym that means "generally recognized as safe." This indicates that, because of its widespread use, garlic is presumed to be safe until proven otherwise. However, keep in mind that most people eat cooked garlic, not raw garlic. Standardized garlic products are more like raw garlic in that they contain intact alliin. Therefore, widespread food use isn't a complete guarantee that the garlic you buy as medicine is completely safe.

> **The FDA places garlic on its GRAS list, an acronym that means "generally recognized as safe."**

Nonetheless, the side effects of various forms of medicinal garlic reported in scientific journals are almost all minor, and they resolve once garlic therapy is discontinued.

There are a few risks sometimes mentioned in association with garlic, but they are largely theoretical, based on possibilities rather than actual evidence. Probably the most serious of these is the potential for garlic to interact with blood-thinning drugs.

Garlic's Excellent Side-Effect Profile: Odor

Garlic produces few side effects. The biggest problem is not a typical side effect at all: odor. Garlic's most commonly reported side effect is annoying rather than dangerous: the smell. Even "odorless" garlic products produce this problem to some extent. Although it is not significant in terms of health, as many as 30% of those who try garlic give it up for this reason.

One double-blind study set out to specifically investigate garlic breath.[61] The study looked at the effects of daily doses of 300 mg, 600 mg, 900 mg, or 1,200 mg of standardized garlic powder. Participants were asked to keep an odor log and record if and when they noticed a garlic smell on their breath or in their sweat.

As you might expect, people noticed more garlic odor, the more garlic they were taking. Daily doses of 900 to 1,200 mg were associated with a 50% incidence of noticeable fragrance. The authors note that this effect frequently prompts individuals to reduce their dose and speculate that participants enrolled in studies may have done so as well, potentially reducing garlic's apparent effectiveness.

However, not everyone dislikes the smell of garlic, and different individuals experience different degrees of odor. People who have trouble with garlic odor might try switching to another kind of garlic product before giving up on it as an herbal medicine.

"Odorless" garlic powder products are not truly odorless, but they do cause little to no immediate garlic breath. The reason is that they don't release allicin until they proceed for a while down the intestinal tract. However, once it is produced, allicin travels through the body and causes odor to arise from the lungs or skin.

People who have trouble with garlic odor might try switching to another kind of garlic product before giving it up altogether.

Thus, while these products are much less smelly than garlic itself, they don't fully eliminate this side effect. Aged garlic may be even better, because it doesn't produce any allicin at all. Such products have not been studied as well as garlic powder standardized to alliin content, but do seem to be effective nonetheless (see Beyond Cholesterol: Garlic's Other Benefits for Your Arteries and How to Take Garlic).

Garlic's Other Side Effects

Participants in garlic studies have reported a few other minor side effects besides odor. However, these are probably not actual problems caused by garlic. In the double-blind placebo-controlled studies of garlic, the incidence of side effects aside from odor was never any higher than what was seen in the placebo group.

Yes, people taking placebo report side effects! It's not uncommon for as many as 20 to 30% of people given placebo treatments to report such problems as headaches, nausea, fatigue, dizziness, and allergic reactions. Just as taking a pill can make you feel better through the power of suggestion, it seems that just the idea of taking a pill is enough to make some people feel sick.

In one study of 261 individuals, less than 1% of those taking garlic reported minor stomach upset, while about 2.5% of those taking placebo experienced the same problem.[62] It is most likely that the stomachaches seen in the garlic group were not truly caused by the garlic, any more than the side effects in the placebo group were caused by placebo.

A large study performed in 1993 evaluated 1,997 individuals to see if taking 900 mg of garlic daily would cause any serious side effects.[63] Studies of this type are called "drug monitoring" studies. They don't involve a placebo group, but simply follow a large group of people for an extended period of time, looking for rare or delayed problems. This study lasted 16 weeks.

Researchers asked study participants about their experiences with side effects at the beginning of the study, and again after 8 and 16 weeks of treatment. No serious side effects were observed. The most common complaint was nausea (6%), followed by dizziness on standing up (1.3%), and allergic reaction to garlic (1.1%). Less than 1% reported other complaints such as bloating, headaches, dizziness at rest, and sweating. However, since there was no placebo group in this study, it can't be determined what proportion of these side effects was real. The major evidence provided by this study is that garlic causes no dangerous side effects.

However, raw garlic appears to be able to cause more side effects than the garlic preparations usually used in studies. Symptoms such as heartburn, upset stomach, headache, flushed skin,

rapid pulse, insomnia, flatulence, and diarrhea have all been reported by people who ate large amounts of fresh garlic. Some
people are particularly intolerant of garlic, and they experience
some gastrointestinal complaints even when they eat just a little.

There have also been several reports of fresh garlic causing
contact *dermatitis* (a rash on the skin).[64–66] As the name im-
plies, this is an allergic condition that appears after touching
garlic. It usually manifests as a red, often scaly rash wherever
the garlic touched, such as the palms of the hands. Most of
these cases occurred in people who handled a lot of raw garlic
on a regular basis: caterers, cooks, farmers, and homemakers.
There are no reports that handling other garlic preparations
can cause this problem.

Garlic can also cause burns when applied directly to the
skin.[67] These usually occur when crushed or cut garlic is left on
the skin for a considerable period of time. Garlic has long been
applied directly to wounds to prevent infections, and physicians
who did so had to use care not to cause a burn (see Garlic and
Modern Medicine). Since you won't be using topical garlic to
lower your cholesterol, you shouldn't encounter this problem.

Garlic's Side Effects Versus
Those of Conventional Medications

How do the side effects of garlic compare with those of cholesterol-lowering medications? Unfortunately, it's difficult to answer this question with certainty. There has been only one
direct comparison of garlic with a standard cholesterol-lowering
medication, and it did not involve the most popular type of cholesterol medication, the statin drugs (see chapter 6, The Statin
Family: Powerful Medications with Few Side Effects).

In this study (see Garlic Versus Conventional Medications),
garlic was compared to the European drug bezafibrate.[68] A
handful of people in each group complained of at least one side
effect. Those in the garlic group mentioned such problems as
reduced appetite, headache, fatigue, and dizziness. Members
of the bezafibrate group reported muscle pain, fatigue, lack of

appetite, and heat discomfort. More than half of those taking garlic reported garlic odor, but none stopped taking it for this reason. This study tells us that garlic is neither better nor worse than bezafibrate with regard to immediate side effects.

In the absence of direct comparative studies, we can consider separate studies and compare the side effects that were reported. For example, we can look at the side effect rate of statin drugs in their studies, and compare this against garlic's side effects in its own studies. However, such comparisons aren't really fair. Side effect incidence varies widely from one study to another, depending on who participates in the study, what kinds of questions the researchers ask, and how researchers interpret responses. Individuals in certain cultures may tend to complain more than others, so it isn't fair to compare a German study of garlic against an American study of a drug. Trying to do so is comparing apples to oranges.

However, it's certainly fair to say at least that garlic seems free of one of the most troubling side effects of cholesterol-lowering drugs: liver inflammation. As many as 1 to 2% of people who take the most popular cholesterol-lowering drugs develop signs of liver problems (see Safety Issues). While only part of this figure is due to the drug itself (people in the placebo group also developed this problem), there is not the slightest hint that garlic causes liver inflammation. Enough people have participated in garlic studies that if this problem were to occur at any significant rate, it would have been noticed. The fact that garlic does not appear to irritate the liver is a real safety plus.

There is one other issue to consider: long-term risk. There are some indications that various cholesterol-lowering medications might increase the risk of cancer (see Safety Issues). There is no evidence that heavy garlic use increases the risk of cancer, and some evidence even suggests that it may help prevent it.[69] In the Nurses' Health study, 41,837 women between the ages of 55 and 69 completed a questionnaire about how frequently they ate certain foods.[70] Researchers followed the women for 5 years and monitored them for cancer. The results showed that women who ate a lot of garlic were 30% less likely to develop colon cancer than those who ate only a little garlic.

Similar evidence has been found in many other studies of this type.[71] (For more information on garlic's possible preventive effect on cancer, see *The Natural Pharmacist: Reducing Cancer Risk.*) Keep in mind, however, that these studies involved dietary garlic, most of which was undoubtedly cooked. Standardized garlic extracts contain many substances not found in cooked garlic, and could conceivably act quite differently. Thus, it isn't really right to assume that garlic has a cancer-preventive effect when taken in the forms used to lower cholesterol.

Toxicity

Toxicity is a slightly different issue from side effects. This term usually refers to a substance's ability to cause severe harm when taken in excessive doses. Many substances can be toxic if you take enough. But some are more toxic than others.

Scientists measure toxicity by determining how large a dose is required to kill 50% of a given group of laboratory animals. This dose is called the "LD_{50}," meaning the lethal dose in 50%.

We know much more about the safety of aged garlic than other forms of garlic. In one study, rats were given up to 2,000 mg/kg of aged garlic extract for a period of 6 months.[72] No toxic symptoms were observed, and examination of organs and tissue found no hidden damage. The only thing that researchers noticed was that rats that were given garlic ate less than the control group. (Maybe garlic should be marketed as a diet aid!)

To put this dose in perspective, consider that the amount given to the rats is equivalent to about 120 to 150 grams/day for an average-sized person. Since the recommended dose of aged garlic is 1 to 7.2 grams daily, you will see that there is a large margin of safety.

However, aged garlic is known to contain virtually no alliin, allicin, or disulfides. It may be that other forms of garlic, such as raw garlic or garlic standardized to alliin, are more toxic. Since there have been no animal toxicity studies on garlic powder standardized to alliin content, we don't really know for sure. This is unfortunate, because this is the most popular type of medicinal garlic.

Aged garlic has also been tested for *genotoxicity* (damage to the genetic material) and *mutagenicity* (ability to cause mutations in the genetic material).[73] The results suggest that garlic doesn't increase the risk of cancer—at least not by damaging or causing mutations in the genes. Unfortunately, once more, there have been no comparable studies of standardized garlic powder.

Garlic and the Blood

Garlic interferes with platelets (which are responsible for blood clotting), and may also help the body to dissolve existing blood clots (see Garlic and Blood Clotting (Hemostasis)). This may mean that garlic can cause excessive bleeding in certain individuals. At present, this remains a theoretical risk, because there have been no reports of excessive bleeding definitely associated with the use of garlic.

In 1990, there was a case report of *spontaneous spinal epidural hematoma* (spontaneous bleeding around the spinal cord) occurring in an 87-year-old man who claimed to be eating four cloves of raw garlic daily. It's not clear whether the garlic really had anything to do with his condition, because in 41% of individuals with this condition, no cause is ever determined. Still, to be on the safe side, certain people should consult a physician before using garlic. In particular, I would certainly recommend caution if you have a bleeding disorder (such as hemophilia). Furthermore, if you are about to have surgery, have just had surgery, or are pregnant and nearly ready to deliver, garlic might not be a good idea.

Surgery and childbirth inevitably involve bleeding, and there has been one report of increased bleeding following TURP surgery (the primary treatment for enlarged prostate gland) in a man who took garlic.[74] While this is a single case report, it is somewhat worrisome. Because you want your blood to clot normally and stop the bleeding, you should avoid taking garlic supplements for 2 weeks or so before surgery or child-birth and during the recovery period.

Drug Interactions

There are no known drug interactions between garlic and conventional medications. This is not to say that they don't occur; but I can say with certainty that none have been reported. It's possible that some interactions have occurred, but that they've been mistaken for side effects of the medication rather than the result of an interaction with garlic.

There are serious concerns that garlic might interact with blood-thinning medications. Some of these medications, such as Coumadin, are rather touchy drugs, and various medications (and even foods) can affect their action. It is very possible that garlic's slight blood-thinning effect could combine with the more powerful effect of such medications and lead to *excessive* thinning of the blood. The results could be dangerous, especially if you were to get in an automobile accident while taking both at once.

It is very possible that garlic's slight blood-thinning effect could combine with the more powerful effect of medications such as Coumadin and lead to bleeding problems.

The most powerful drugs in this category are Coumadin (warfarin) and heparin. Aspirin and Trental (pentoxifylline) also interfere with blood clotting to a much more modest extent. If you are taking any medications of this type, you should consult your physician before taking garlic. Furthermore, a few natural substances are also mild blood thinners, such as the herb ginkgo and vitamin E. Conceivably, bleeding problems might develop when you combine these treatments, although no such problems have been reported.

Based on indirect evidence, people in certain medical circumstances might want to be especially cautious in using garlic.

Pemphigus

Pemphigus is a rare autoimmune disease that involves the skin and mucous membranes. Characterized by large, fluid-filled blisters and thickening of the skin, it most often occurs in people between 30 and 60 years of age, and it can be fatal.

A certain chemical compound called a *thiol group* can worsen pemphigus. Since garlic contains an active thiol group, there are some concerns that it might potentially cause a similar problem. For the same reason, people with this disease are cautioned to avoid other foods in the garlic family, such as leeks, onions, shallots, and chives.

Organ Transplants

At high doses, garlic has been shown to activate certain cells of the immune system called natural killer (NK) cells.[75,76] These are a type of white blood cell that patrols our bodies looking for bacteria, viruses, and other invaders, and helps to remove them. People who receive organ transplants don't want their natural killer cells activated, because these cells can cause organ transplant rejection. NK cells may attack the new organ as if it were an enemy. Organ transplant recipients are usually treated with drugs that suppress NK cells—as well as other parts of the immune system—to keep the transplanted organ safe. Garlic could conceivably reverse this suppression.

Diabetes

Weak evidence suggests that garlic may lower blood sugar (glucose). If true, this could make it paradoxically both helpful and dangerous for people with diabetes. The danger would come if garlic caused a sudden or unanticipated drop in blood-sugar levels (hypoglycemia). People with diabetes are often skirting the edge of hypoglycemia, and a sudden drop in blood sugar can be dangerous. On the other hand, if garlic has a mild, gentle effect of reducing blood sugar, it could conceivably play a helpful role in maintaining a healthy blood-sugar level.

However, there's not much evidence to suggest that garlic actually reduces blood-sugar levels. Some animal studies have found this effect, while others have not, and it has not been seen in human studies. Still, to be on the safe side, if you have diabetes and are considering whether or not to use garlic, consult your physician to assess the potential risk of altering your blood-sugar levels.

Long-Term Risks

A question people often ask about herbs is whether it is safe to take them for many years. This is a legitimate concern because many drugs cause problems that only become evident after a long period of use, and herbs could conceivably do the same thing. For more information on the positive results of two garlic-related long-term studies, see Does Garlic Reduce Deaths from Heart Disease? and Garlic's Side Effects Versus Those of Conventional Medications. These studies suggest that garlic may help prevent heart attacks and reduce cancer risk.

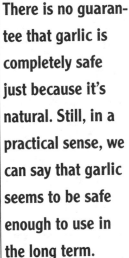

There is no guarantee that garlic is completely safe just because it's natural. Still, in a practical sense, we can say that garlic seems to be safe enough to use in the long term.

Garlic is probably safe even when taken for a while. Still, we don't know absolutely for sure. Of course, a very ancient and worldwide tradition of use has failed to turn up any health problems associated with long-term garlic use, but this doesn't mean that there couldn't be rare, hidden, subtle, or occasional side effects that simply haven't yet been noticed.

The reality is that the same lack of knowledge prevails for virtually all medical therapies. The only absolutely foolproof way to determine whether or not long-term harm exists would be to take two identical populations, give one-half the drug and the other half placebo, and keep the experiment going for decades. If after 50 years or so, no problems cropped up in the treated group, one could then conclude that a treatment was probably safe in the long run.

Obviously, such an experiment has never been done—for drugs, herbs, vaccinations, food preservatives, or foods. Thus, the long-term safety of all treatments must be regarded as not yet rigorously established.

Some people feel that because garlic is a natural herb, it is more likely than a drug to be safe in the long run. However, this is more of an emotional statement than a rational one. Numerous herbs have been shown to be potentially toxic, including comfrey and chaparral. For that matter, fatty foods appear to be carcinogenic. In other words, there is no guarantee that garlic is completely safe just because it's natural. Still, in a practical sense, long-term garlic use is probably safe, and it may even be beneficial.

Garlic and Pregnant or Nursing Women

There haven't been any animal or human studies that specifically examined whether standardized garlic powder affects embryos, fetuses, or young children. Therefore, safety cannot be assured for pregnant or nursing women.

Garlic is one of many foods that may cause colic in babies when their nursing mothers eat it. However, obstetricians do not warn pregnant women to avoid eating raw garlic, and no bad occurrences have been documented among women who have done so. It seems unlikely that standardized garlic powder presents any greater risks than raw garlic, but we cannot guarantee this. Finally, garlic probably shouldn't be used in the weeks prior to labor and delivery (see Garlic and the Blood).

Other Supplements for High Cholesterol

Many over-the-counter supplements are available that can help lower your cholesterol. Red yeast rice, gugulipid, pantethine, and niacin are all supplements that seem to have a positive impact on lipid levels. Vitamin C and tocotrienols also may be helpful, although the evidence is somewhat contradictory.

These products are often used in conjunction with garlic therapy in the hopes of producing a more powerful cholesterol-lowering effect. While there is little research using multiple supplements to lower cholesterol, in practice it appears that combination therapy may produce better results than any one treatment alone.

Red Yeast Rice: A Promising New Herbal Treatment for High Cholesterol

Red yeast rice seems to be one of the most promising natural treatments on the market for lowering cholesterol. This product is a traditional Chinese food that is made by fermenting a type of yeast called *Monascus purpureus* over rice. Under the traditional name *Hong Qu*, red yeast rice has been used in China as a food and medicinal substance since at least A.D. 800.

It is used to treat indigestion, diarrhea, and abdominal pain. Today, it is also used in winemaking and as a food coloring. It was recently discovered that this ancient Chinese preparation contains more than 11 naturally occurring substances closely related to approved statin drugs, the leading cholesterol-lowering drugs on the market (see The Statin Family: Powerful Medications with Few Side Effects in chapter 6). Based on this discovery and other related studies, red yeast rice has become a popular over-the-counter cholesterol-reducing agent.

Red yeast rice contains more than 11 naturally occurring chemicals in the statin drug family.

One product of the fermentation process of red yeast rice is *mevinolin*, an HMG-CoA reductase inhibitor that is similar to the synthetically produced lovastatin. Other constituents produced from fermentation include flavonoids and unsaturated fatty acids, which may also contribute to the cholesterol-lowering effect.

What Is the Scientific Evidence for Red Yeast Rice?

Of the more than two dozen clinical studies of red yeast rice using human participants, two were conducted in the U.S., and the rest were conducted in China. In the following pages I discuss the two most recent studies in detail.

The U.S. study was a randomized, double-blind, placebo-controlled trial conducted at the UCLA School of Medicine.[1] Cholestin was found to significantly improve the levels of total cholesterol, LDL cholesterol, and, to a lesser extent, triglycerides. Only very small or no improvements in cholesterol levels occurred in the placebo group. In fact, triglycerides increased slightly in this group.

The 12-week trial involved 83 healthy participants (46 men and 37 women aged 34-78 years). One group of 42 participants was given the recommended Cholestin daily dose (2 capsules twice daily). Another group of 41 participants took a placebo capsule containing rice powder. Both groups were instructed to follow the American Heart Association Step I diet. After 8 weeks on Cholestin, average total cholesterol (mg/dL) fell from 250 to 208 (17%). During the same time period, average LDL cholesterol (the bad kind) decreased from 173 to 134 (22.4%) and average triglycerides dropped from 133 to 118 (11%). After 12 weeks, the decreases in total cholesterol and LDL cholesterol were maintained, while triglycerides went back up about 6 mg/dL to 124, so that the net decrease in triglycerides was 6.7%. HDL cholesterol (the good kind), which averaged 50 mg/dL at the beginning of the study, did not change during the 12 weeks. Meanwhile, the placebo group experienced only minor changes.

The researchers concluded that red yeast rice significantly reduces total cholesterol, LDL cholesterol, and triglycerides compared to placebo and provides a new, novel, food-based approach to lowering cholesterol in the general population.

The Chinese study[2] found even greater improvements in cholesterol than the UCLA trial. Like the UCLA trial, this was a randomized, double-blind, placebo-controlled trial. It examined the effects of a more concentrated form of Cholestin in elderly patients. In the 8-week trial, one group of 35 patients took 1.2 g daily of red yeast rice while another group of 35 took a placebo pill. The red yeast rice formulation used was a more concentrated version than usual. The lead author, Joseph Chang, Ph.D., reported that Cholestin reduced total cholesterol by almost 26%, LDL cholesterol by 33%, and triglycerides by 20%. Chang said HDL cholesterol was not measured in this study. These improvements were substantially greater than those found in the placebo group.

Evidence suggests that red yeast rice can lower blood cholesterol.

Researchers concluded that the use of this form of red yeast rice as a dietary supplement was safe in the elderly and that it may represent an effective, novel way to manage the high levels of cholesterol and triglycerides that influence cardiovascular health.

Dosage

The standard dose of red yeast rice is 600 mg twice a day. Red yeast rice is widely available in capsule form at pharmacies and health-food stores.

Because it contains ingredients similar to those in statin drugs, red yeast rice should be used under medical supervision.

The product is standardized to contain 0.4% total HMG-CoA reductase inhibitors, which at the recommended dose would deliver about 5 mg of these chemicals. This is a very small dose compared to the average dose of the conventional HMG-CoA reductase inhibitor lovastatin, for example, which is 40 mg. Thus, there is a very real question whether the dose in red yeast rice is high enough to account for 100% of the benefits seen in the research. There may be other important constituents in red yeast rice as well, but more research is needed to answer this question.

Safety Issues

While there have been no serious adverse reactions reported in the studies of red yeast rice, some minor side effects have been reported in very small numbers. The most common side effects are heartburn, bloating, and dizziness, and as discussed in Safety Issues with Garlic, they are quite consistent with the types of problems often reported by those given placebo.

Formal toxicity studies in rats and mice found no toxic effects even with doses equivalent to 125 times the normal human dose given for 3 months, according to unpublished information on file with one of the manufacturers of red yeast rice.[3]

It is important to note that because red yeast contains ingredients similar to those in the statin drugs, there is a very real possibility that it can cause the same adverse side effects seen with the statins. These include elevated liver enzymes, damage to muscles and kidneys, and possible increased risk of cancer. Although these side effects have not been reported, it's possible that they may occur, which is one reason you should take red yeast rice only under a doctor's supervision.

Warning: There are no known drug interactions with red yeast rice. However, statin drugs should not be combined with niacin, erythromycin, cyclosporine, fibrates, or other statin drugs (see The Statin Family: Powerful Medications with Few Side Effects). The same cautions may apply to red yeast rice. Similarly, this product should not be taken by pregnant or nursing mothers or those with severe liver or kidney disease, except with a physician's advice.

Gugulipid: A Traditional Indian Herb

Gugulipid is the standardized extract derived from the bark of the Mukul myrrh tree *(Commiphora mukul)*, a small, thorny tree native to India and Arabia. This substance has been used for thousands of years as part of a traditional Indian medical system called *Ayurveda*. It appears to be able to reduce total cholesterol by about 12% and LDL ("bad") cholesterol by 12 to 17%.

What Is the Scientific Evidence for Gugulipid?

Animal and human studies have found gugulipid effective at lowering cholesterol. One double-blind placebo-controlled study investigated the effect of

Gugulipid appears to be able to reduce total cholesterol by about 12% and LDL ("bad") cholesterol by 12 to 17%.

dietary modification and gugulipid on cholesterol levels in 61 people.[4] Half of the group received 100 mg of gugulipid and the others received placebo. All of them were put on a fruit- and vegetable-enriched diet.

After 24 weeks, the gugulipid group's lipid profiles had changed significantly. Total cholesterol fell by 11.7%, LDL ("bad") cholesterol fell by 12.5%, and triglycerides fell by 12%. HDL ("good") cholesterol remained unchanged. There was no significant change in the placebo group. In this study, gugulipid clearly worked better than placebo.

Another double-blind placebo-controlled crossover study compared the effects of gugulipid with the fibric acid derivative drug clofibrate (see Fibric Acid Derivatives: Better for Treating High Triglyceride Levels).[5] Two hundred and thirty-three people were enrolled in the study. The average total cholesterol was 258 mg/dL in the gugulipid group and 281 mg/dL in the clofibrate group. Both groups took 500 mg 3 times a day of either gugulipid or clofibrate for a period of 12 weeks. Afterward, there was a brief washout period (during which neither group received any treatment), and then the two groups' treatments were switched for an additional 8 weeks.

Gugulipid is a substance that has been used for thousands of years as part of a traditional Indian medical system called Ayurveda.

In this study, gugulipid was more effective than clofibrate at improving cholesterol levels. Although clofibrate decreased total cholesterol slightly more than gugulipid (15% versus 13%), gugulipid had more of an effect on LDL cholesterol, which is probably more important than total cholesterol. LDL dropped 17% in those on gugulipid versus a 13% decrease in the clofibrate group. HDL also increased significantly in the gugulipid group (16%), while the clofibrate group did not see a change that was statistically significant. Other studies in humans have also found gugulipid effective at lowering cholesterol.[6,7]

The main constituents of gugulipid are substances called *guggulsterones.* Both E-guggulsterone and Z-guggulsterone are believed (but not proven) to be the active ingredients. We don't know how gugulipid works. One study in rats suggests that guggulsterones cause the liver to remove LDL from the blood.[8]

Dosage

Most of the clinical studies have used a product standardized to contain 5 to 10% guggulsterones, taken at a dose of 500 mg 3 times a day. The course of treatment should be 3 to 6 months. Gugulipid is widely available in pharmacies and health-food stores.

Safety Issues

Based on animal toxicity studies, gugulipid appears to be quite safe. In 6-month toxicity studies in rats, monkeys, and beagles, gugulipid showed no adverse effects.[9,10] In a toxicity study using mice, the LD30 (the dose needed to kill 30% of the mice) was 1,600 mg/kg, or roughly 50 times the recommended dose.[11] However, there haven't been any long-term safety studies in humans.

Gugulipid occasionally causes minor side effects such as nausea, headache, and belching. There are no known interactions between gugulipid and drugs. Animal studies suggest that gugulipid may be safe during pregnancy, but again, human evidence is lacking. Safety in young children, pregnant or nursing women, or those with severe liver or kidney disease has not been established.

Pantethine: Particularly Effective for Elevated Triglycerides

Pantethine is closely related to pantothenic acid, or vitamin B_5. The name is derived from the Greek word *pantos,* which means "everywhere." Indeed, vitamin B_5 can be found in virtually every type of food. It is a major component of a molecule called *coenzyme A* (CoA), which is important because it is involved in many biochemical pathways and responsible for the transport of fats in and out of cells.

What Is the Scientific Evidence for Pantethine?

According to a few small studies, pantethine can strikingly lower triglyceride levels and improve total and LDL cholesterol. For reasons that are not clear, vitamin B_5 itself has not been found to work.

One double-blind placebo-controlled study examined 29 individuals with elevated cholesterol and triglycerides.[12] Participants were given either 900 mg of pantethine or placebo daily for 8 weeks, then treatments were switched for an additional 8 weeks. The results showed that pantethine could reduce total cholesterol and LDL by about 13.5%. Even more impressively, triglycerides went down by 30%.

> According to a few small studies, pantethine can strikingly lower triglyceride levels and improve total and LDL cholesterol.

Another double-blind placebo-controlled study of 29 people with an average total cholesterol of 278 mg/dL found comparable results with 1,200 mg of pantethine daily.[13] Some natural medicine authorities suggest that pantethine may be particularly useful as a cholesterol-lowering supplement for people who have diabetes. The reason for this is that there is concern that some other cholesterol-lowering agents (specifically niacin and, theoretically, garlic) can affect blood sugar levels. A few studies have used pantethine in those who have diabetes and have found no changes in insulin or blood-glucose levels.[14,15] However, in reality, no study in humans has found garlic to affect blood-sugar levels either, so this "advantage" may not amount to much.

Pantethine is believed to lower cholesterol by inhibiting HMG-CoA reductase, an effect similar to that of the statin drugs (see The Statin Family: Powerful Medications with Few Side Effects).[16] Another theory is that pantethine causes the body to "burn" fat faster, but this has not been clearly shown.

Dosage

The recommended dose of pantethine is 300 mg 3 times daily. You should see results within about 1 month. Unfortunately, pantethine is expensive. Because of its high price, I recommend pantethine as an alternative only after other less-costly methods have failed to work for you.

Safety Issues

Pantethine appears to be a safe supplement. One long-term study gave 24 individuals 900 mg of pantethine daily for 1 year without any problems.[17] Formal animal toxicity studies have not been done, but there have been no reports of adverse effects in any of the human studies on pantethine. There are no known drug interactions with pantethine. Safety in pregnant or nursing women or those with severe liver or kidney disease has not been established.

Vitamin C: Possibly Helpful for High Cholesterol

Vitamin C, also known as *ascorbic acid*, is an important antioxidant nutrient that plays many different roles in the body. Our bodies don't manufacture vitamin C, so we have to get it from our food. Fortunately, many foods are high in vitamin C; not only oranges and lemons, but also green peppers, potatoes, and many other fresh fruits and vegetables.

In the past, people who received poor nourishment, such as sailors, developed severe deficiencies in vitamin C and the symptoms of a disease known as *scurvy.* Scurvy is a breakdown of connective tissue. Its symptoms include weakness, loss of teeth, reopening of old wounds, and even death. Fortunately, scurvy is rarely seen anymore.

Besides preventing scurvy, vitamin C supplements may have numerous other health benefits, including reducing the severity and duration of the common cold. Numerous studies have evaluated vitamin C to determine whether it can lower cholesterol levels. However, the results have been somewhat inconclusive.

What Is the Scientific Evidence for Vitamin C?

More than 21 clinical studies on humans have looked at vitamin C's effects on atherosclerosis. Unfortunately, only three of these were properly designed, double-blind placebo-controlled studies. To make matters even less clear, the results of these three double-blind studies conflict. In fact, their results were so different that no one is sure how to make sense of them.

One group of researchers attempted to put together all the human studies of vitamin C and cholesterol in a meta-analysis, but the inconsistency in number of participants, dose used, and length of the studies made it impossible to get accurate results.[18] The bottom line is that although vitamin C has been the object of numerous studies regarding its effects on cholesterol, we really don't know whether it is effective.

Dosage

A dosage of 250 to 500 mg of vitamin C per day may be adequate, though higher doses are often recommended.

Safety Issues

In general, vitamin C appears to be quite safe. The most common side effect of too much vitamin C is diarrhea and abdominal cramping. This usually occurs in people taking more than 1 g of vitamin C per day, and resolves once the dose is cut back. To avoid this problem, take vitamin C in divided doses (for example, 100 mg 3 times a day versus 300 mg at once) or use a buffered form. Starting with a low dose and increasing the dose slowly may also help prevent this problem.

People susceptible to kidney stones are also sometimes cautioned not to take vitamin C, although this recommendation has been disputed.[19]

People with a disease called *hemochromatosis* (excessive storage of iron in the body) or other iron metabolism diseases should use caution when supplementing with vitamin C. Vitamin C increases the body's absorption of iron and can exacerbate the problem.

People who take large doses of vitamin C regularly should not stop abruptly. Finally, vitamin C may cause false readings on certain lab tests, such as occult blood (blood in the stool) and some urine tests. If your doctor orders any lab tests for you, make sure he or she knows that you are taking vitamin C.

If your doctor orders any lab tests for you, make sure he or she knows that you are taking vitamin C.

There are no known drug interactions with vitamin C. The safety of vitamin C in pregnancy is unknown, although no adverse effects have been reported. According to Alan Gaby, M.D., an expert in the field of nutritional medicine, breast-fed infants may experience signs of colic if mothers ingest large quantities of vitamin C.

Tocotrienols: Promising for High Cholesterol

Tocotrienols are naturally occurring substances that are forms of vitamin E and that may offer some benefit in lowering your cholesterol. They are found in high amounts in palm oil and rice bran oil.

What Is the Scientific Evidence for Tocotrienols?

The few controlled trials on tocotrienols that have been performed in humans have produced varied findings. One researcher evaluated a special mixture of tocotrienols plus vitamin E (alpha-tocopherol) in a double-blind placebo-controlled study of 41 people with high cholesterol levels.[20] Total cholesterol fell by 16% and LDL cholesterol fell by 23% in the treatment group, compared to 7% and 11%, respectively, in the placebo group.

Like garlic, pantethine, and the statin drugs, tocotrienols seem to inhibit the enzyme HMG-CoA reductase, at least in test-tube studies.[21] However, we don't know if this is what tocotrienols actually do when people take them orally. More research needs to be done before we can pinpoint with confidence the mechanism for tocotrienols' effect on cholesterol.

Furthermore, another controlled trial found that the same branded tocotrienol mixture used in the study just mentioned may help protect against atherosclerosis, but surprisingly, showed no benefit in lowering cholesterol.[22] Fifty individuals with atherosclerosis involving the brain were followed over 18 months. Of the 25 treated participants, plaque deposits appeared to improve in seven and to progress in two. None of the 25 participants in the control group showed improvement and 10 showed progression. But there was no change in cholesterol levels in either group. This directly contradicts the first study and leaves us somewhat in the dark as to whether tocotrienols actually work. Larger studies are needed to help sort out this tangle.

One study suggests that tocotrienols may work better when they are not combined with vitamin E (alphatocopherol). But this doesn't mean that you should throw out your vitamin E supplements and switch to rice bran oil. There is very good evidence that vitamin E supplements can help prevent heart disease. This evidence is much stronger than what we presently know regarding tocotrienols. For more information on vitamin E and its apparent ability to reduce the chance of developing heart disease, see *The Natural Pharmacist: Heart Disease Prevention.*

Dosage

We don't know enough about tocotrienols to determine the best therapeutic dose. A dose frequently recommended is one to two 25 mg capsules daily. However, in one of the studies described above, a 220 mg tocotrienol mixture was used.

Safety Issues

There have not been any reported side effects or signs of toxicity at the doses used in the studies, but formal safety studies on tocotrienols have not been done. Maximum safe doses have not been determined for pregnant or nursing women or those with severe kidney or liver disease.

Additional Proposed Treatments for High Cholesterol

Several other natural substances have been proposed as treatments for high cholesterol. The major substances are listed below.

Soy

Soy foods are going mainstream. The U.S. Food and Drug Administration allows manufacturers of foods containing soy to label their products with the claim that, when consumed in combination with a healthful diet, soy products may lower cholesterol and reduce the risk of heart disease. The scientific evidence for this position is quite impressive. Studies suggest that using soy protein instead of animal protein can lower total cholesterol by an average of 9%, lower LDL ("bad") cholesterol by 13%, and lower triglycerides by 10.5%.[23]

The amount of soy necessary to reduce cholesterol appears to be approximately 25 g daily—approximately two servings of tofu or two cups of soy milk. If you like the taste of soy products such as tofu and tempeh, you're in luck. Soy is one of the most versatile foods in the world. In centuries of traditional use in Asia, tofu has been braised, stir-fried, steamed, and deep-fried in a variety of ways. Today, you can also buy tofu hot dogs, tofu burgers, soy "cheese," and tempeh "turkey" drumsticks.

Yet soy seems to be one of those foods that is loved by some and hated passionately by others. If you can't imagine eating "soysage" instead of sausage in your spaghetti sauce, you can still benefit from trading some of the meat in your diet for plant-based protein. If eating meat is important to you, try replacing half the meat in your stew with lentils or barley. If you've never put beans in your chili before, try it. Use just a little meat to flavor split pea or bean soup.

Fish Oil

While it is very important to cut down on saturated fat in your diet, certain fats may actually be healthy for you.

Fish contain omega-3 fatty acids, a form of polyunsaturated fat that may be protective against heart disease. Omega-3 fatty acids are "essential fatty acids" that are not made by the body and must be supplied by the diet or by supplements. Interest in them began when it was found that natives of northern Canada who lived extensively on fish had few heart attacks despite a very high fat intake. Subsequent studies, however, have come to mixed conclusions.[24,25] It appears that the omega-3 fatty acids produce little effect on total cholesterol levels, but significantly decrease triglycerides. They may slightly raise LDL cholesterol, but this effect is usually temporary.[26] Fish oil may also help prevent blood clots, lower blood pressure, and decrease homocysteine levels. (Homocysteine is another suspected risk factor for atherosclerosis. See Atherosclerosis and High Cholesterol.)[27] The bottom line is that it is unclear whether fish oil is beneficial for atherosclerosis and heart disease.[28,29]

Fish oil appears to be safe. Contrary to some reports, it does not seem to increase bleeding or affect blood-sugar control in people with diabetes.[30] For more information on fish oil, see *The Natural Pharmacist: Natural Health Bible.* Flax oil has been suggested as an alternative to fish oil.[31] However, there is no evidence that flax oil is effective, and it does not lower triglycerides.

Aortic Glycosaminoglycans (GAGs)

Aortic glycosaminoglycans (GAGs) are substances found in high concentrations in the walls of the arteries. Taking GAG supplements may slow the progression of atherosclerosis and possibly reduce cholesterol levels, although we are not sure how.

In a recent controlled (but not double-blind) study, a group of men with early hardening of the coronary arteries was given 200 mg per day of GAGs.[32] After 18 months, the layering of the vessel lining was 7.5 times greater in the untreated group than in the GAG group, a significant difference. While a double-blind study is necessary to confirm these benefits, this research does suggest that aortic GAGs can significantly slow the progression of atherosclerosis.

The same benefit has been seen in animal studies.[33] According to one controlled study, aortic GAGs may also reduce the chance of heart attacks.[34] We don't know how aortic GAGs work. There is some evidence that they can reduce cholesterol levels and thin the blood.[35,36] However, more research is necessary.

L-Carnitine

Another supplement that might show some benefit is L-carnitine. L-carnitine is an amino acid that the body uses to turn fat into energy. It is not normally considered an essential nutrient, since the body can manufacture all it needs. However, supplemental L-carnitine may improve the ability of certain tissues to produce energy. This has led to the use of L-carnitine in various muscle diseases as well as heart conditions.

Weak evidence suggests that L-carnitine may be able to improve cholesterol and triglyceride levels.[37] Since L-carnitine is very expensive, and there is little evidence as yet that it works, I recommend using other more proven and cost-effective therapies to reduce your cholesterol.

Calcium

Calcium supplements may occasionally lower cholesterol.[38] A typical nutritional dose is 1,000 to 1,200 mg daily. Calcium is probably more useful as a treatment for osteoporosis. See *The Natural Pharmacist: Natural Health Bible* for more information—including what type of calcium to purchase and a discussion of safety issues.

Lecithin

Although there is a widespread belief that lecithin can lower cholesterol, a recent small, double-blind study of 23 men with high cholesterol levels found that lecithin treatment had no significant effects on total blood cholesterol, triglycerides, HDL cholesterol, LDL cholesterol, or lipoprotein(a).[39] There is little good positive evidence to set against this negative study.

Combination Therapy

What about combining therapies? It seems natural to expect that mixing two or more cholesterol-lowering treatments might produce better results than using garlic alone. According to a holistic physician, Debra Brammer, N.D., "Most patients benefit from combination therapy, but the results may vary considerably. In two people with the same cholesterol level, one may drop 60 points and the other, only 2." This is not surprising, since each person's high cholesterol levels may not be due to exactly the same combination of physiological factors.

Dr. Brammer also cautions that herbs and supplements are only part of the picture. "If a patient isn't eating a healthy diet and exercising, his or her cholesterol doesn't usually change as much as the cholesterol of someone who has made lifestyle changes. The whole person needs to be addressed to get the best results."

We have no research evidence as yet that can tell us just how effective these combination approaches really are. Nonetheless, combining treatments is a logical approach, and one that is frequently used in conventional medicine as well.

Keep in mind that lowering cholesterol is only one part of the picture. There are many ways you can reduce your risk of heart disease. For more information on this complex subject, see *The Natural Pharmacist: Heart Disease Prevention.*

Niacin and
High Cholesterol

N iacin is a water-soluble vitamin, also known as vitamin B_3, that serves many functions in our bodies. It interacts with more than 200 enzymes that help our bodies metabolize fats and sugars and produce energy. Niacin can be found in most animal products, such as liver and other organ meats, poultry, and fish, but it is also found in many plant sources like sesame and sunflower seeds, whole grains, red chili peppers, nuts (especially peanuts, almonds, and pine nuts), and avocados.

Technically, niacin is a nonessential vitamin, meaning that we can live without getting it in our diet. Our bodies are able to make it from another common nutrient, the amino acid *tryptophan*, along with the help of vitamins B_1, B_2, B_6, and C, as well as iron. Nonetheless, most people get plenty of already-formed niacin from the foods they eat, and there is an official minimum daily requirement that will "cover" your niacin needs even if other nutrients are missing.

Niacin can also lower cholesterol. When used for this purpose, it must be taken in amounts much higher than what is manufactured by the body or found in food. This use of niacin was discovered many decades ago, and at one time niacin was the most commonly used conventional treatment for high cholesterol.

Visit Us at TNP.com

The U.S. National Cholesterol Education Program (NCEP) considers niacin to be in the same league as the lipid-lowering drugs discussed in chapter 6. NCEP further suggests that niacin is especially valuable in treating high cholesterol in individuals with low HDL cholesterol, and in those with both high cholesterol and high triglycerides.

Since the advent of the statin drugs, however, most physicians have stopped using niacin. This is due in part to the fact that the statin drugs have shown to be more effective in reducing both total cholesterol and LDL ("bad") cholesterol levels. Niacin has also been associated with annoying (as well as potentially dangerous) side effects. Nevertheless, it is still a highly effective treatment for high cholesterol that is safe if used properly, and is particularly effective at raising HDL ("good") cholesterol levels.

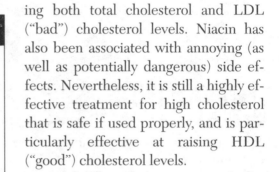

Not only does niacin improve cholesterol levels, like some statin drugs, niacin has also been shown to improve overall mortality.

Not only can niacin improve cholesterol levels, it has been shown to improve overall mortality.[1] Additionally, niacin is one of the few treatments that can dramatically improve HDL ("good") cholesterol levels.

What Is the Scientific Evidence for Niacin?

There is very strong scientific evidence supporting the use of niacin. Unlike garlic, it is widely used in conventional medicine, and niacin has been approved by the FDA.

Several well-designed double-blind placebo-controlled studies have found that niacin reduced total cholesterol by 10 to 25% and reduced triglycerides by as much as 50%.[2–5] Additionally, niacin has been shown to elevate HDL cholesterol by as much as 30%. Niacin also lowers levels of lipoprotein(a)—another risk factor for atherosclerosis—by about 35%.

Niacin: Diet Versus Supplements

Many foods provide high amounts of niacin. The best sources include brewer's yeast; rice bran; wheat bran; peanuts; organ meats, such as liver; and certain types of fish, such as trout, halibut, swordfish, and salmon. Other good sources of niacin are whole grains, wheat germ, pine nuts, sunflower seeds, and split peas.

The U.S. recommended daily allowance (RDA) for niacin for an adult is between 15 and 20 mg daily. Since many foods provide between 7 and 38 mg per 3.5-ounce portion of the food, meeting the RDA requirement typically is not a problem.

However, it is unlikely that you could achieve high enough doses in your diet to get the therapeutic effect. For example, peanuts contain about 16 mg of niacin per 3.5-ounce portion. If you consider that the dose of niacin required to lower cholesterol is about 1,500 mg daily, then you would have to eat almost 328 ounces of peanuts each day, which is about 20 pounds of peanuts! I doubt most people would be able to eat 140 pounds of peanuts each week (not to mention afford buying such large quantities). You really have to take niacin supplements if you wish to use it to improve your cholesterol levels.

Other studies have compared niacin with statin drugs, the most effective and widely used conventional treatments for high cholesterol. These studies have consistently shown that the statin drugs are more effective than niacin when it comes to reducing total cholesterol, but that niacin is more effective in lowering triglycerides and lipoprotein(a) and raising HDL ("good") cholesterol. Also, niacin's effect on total cholesterol tends to become stronger over longer periods of time, suggesting that taken regularly, niacin might be even more effective in reducing cholesterol than the studies have found.

How Does Niacin Work?

As with garlic and many other treatments for high cholesterol, we don't really know how niacin works. Laboratory research has suggested a couple of different theories to explain how niacin lowers cholesterol.

> **Niacin is a highly effective treatment for high cholesterol, and it is safe if used properly.**

One theory is that niacin affects the release of fats into the bloodstream by altering the function of a crucial enzyme.[6] Another theory is that niacin specifically blocks a process that removes HDL from the blood. As you may recall, HDL is believed to help protect arteries from the damaging effects of other forms of cholesterol.[7]

However, as none of these theories has been tested in humans, at this point they're only theoretical speculation.

Dosage

The adult recommended intake of niacin is 19 mg for most adult men and 15 mg for most adult women. Cholesterol-lowering doses are much higher, up to 4,000 mg daily.

When using it to reduce cholesterol levels, you should start niacin at a low dose and gradually increase it over several weeks. For example, begin with 50 to 100 mg 3 times daily taken with or just after meals. Increase the dose 100 to 250 mg every 7 to 14 days. According to one study, a minimum dose of 1,000 mg a day is necessary to get the cholesterol-lowering effect with niacin,[8] but many people require somewhat more. A typical dose is 500 to 1,000 mg 3 times daily. Dosages up to 6 to 9 g have been used, but the larger the dose, the greater the risk of side effects.

Warning: Don't take niacin in cholesterol-lowering doses without medical supervision. At those high doses, niacin is a drug, not a dietary supplement. Keep in mind that even the starting dose of niacin is about ten times more than you need for good nutrition. While you're on niacin therapy, your doctor will want to periodically check your blood liver enzymes to head off any possible liver toxicity—niacin's most serious potential side effect.

The first thing you will notice within 15 minutes to 2 hours of taking niacin is its most common side effect; a skin reaction called *flushing.* Knowing in advance that it's not dangerous does not make it any more comfortable. Prepare for your face and body to turn a shade of red, along with heat sensations, tingling, headache, and itching. You may experience one or more of these symptoms.

To minimize flushing, it's best to build up slowly, starting with a moderate dose and increasing it over several weeks.

In order to reduce flushing, it's best to build up slowly, starting with a moderate dose and increasing it over several weeks. I recommend starting with 250 mg 3 times a day for the first week or two, and then building up. Taking aspirin about 30 minutes before niacin can also inhibit the flushing effect. One study showed that taking 325 mg of aspirin before taking niacin reduced flushing, itching, and tingling by as much as 58%.[9] Aspirin inhibits chemicals in the body called *prostaglandins,* which are responsible for the flushing and perhaps some of the other symptoms. Consult your doctor before starting on aspirin or other similar medication in conjunction with niacin.

Types of Niacin

Another thing to consider when taking niacin is the form you use. Currently, there are three forms of niacin that lower cholesterol, but only two of them are sold over the counter. They are ordinary, immediate-release niacin, "flush-free" developed in Europe *(inositol hexaniacinate),* and slow-release niacin.

Most of the scientific research has been on immediate-release niacin. This is the type you are likely to find at your local pharmacy or health-food store. It is definitely effective and very inexpensive.

Inositol hexaniacinate, also called "flush-free" niacin, was developed in Europe as an alternative to standard niacin. It appears to produce less flushing than regular niacin,[10] but flushing still does occur. Inositol hexaniacinate is also said to be safer for the liver, but this hasn't been proven. This "alternative" form of niacin has been suggested as a treatment for other conditions as well.

> **Niacinamide has many nutritional benefits, but it doesn't lower cholesterol. Be careful to read the labels of the different niacin products to make sure that you get the right form.**

Slow-release niacin is available only by prescription. It produces less flushing, but it is more likely to cause liver inflammation than ordinary immediate-release niacin.

Make sure not to buy *niacinamide* by mistake. As a low dose supplement for general nutrition, niacinamide is identical to niacin, and doesn't cause flushing. But high dose niacinamide does not seem to lower cholesterol.

Be careful to read the labels of the different niacin products to make sure that you get just the form you want.

Safety Issues

So far, you've heard all the good news about niacin. But it also has a downside. Niacin was once a leading conventional treatment for high cholesterol, but it was largely abandoned in favor of the statin drugs. One main reason for this was that niacin produces a number of uncomfortable minor side effects, and some

John's Story

John, 63, was very conscious about his health, and he wanted to get it under control right away before any future problems developed. His cholesterol was moderately high, at 235 mg/dL. John's diet was already good; he was eating a good balance of nutrients and getting plenty of fiber. He and his wife were avid walkers who spent at least 30 minutes almost every night walking in their neighborhood. Since he already had the diet and exercise pieces of his health taken care of, he began taking a standardized garlic extract and added garlic to his diet as well.

After about 3 months, John's cholesterol level had only dropped slightly, to 230 mg/dL. John wanted to try a more aggressive approach, and began taking niacin in addition to the garlic, at a dose of 250 mg 3 times a day to start, and gradually working up to twice that dosage. John reported that he had noticed the flushing at first, but then it had subsided. He had no other side effects. Six weeks later, his cholesterol had fallen to 194 mg/dL and his HDL had increased by 20%. There has been no sign of liver problems throughout the course of his treatment.

potentially serious risks associated with a particular "slow-release" form of niacin. The side effects can be troublesome enough to discourage some people from taking niacin. Nonetheless, if you use the proper form of niacin at the right dose, you can often avoid these problems.

Side Effects

The most common side effect is "flushing," as described in Dosage. This effect occurs in as many as 50% of people who try niacin. Flushing is not dangerous, but it can be uncomfortable and annoying. Fortunately, it seems to decrease over time as the body gets used to its daily dose of niacin. Flushing can also be increased by alcohol consumption as well as by the alcohol-deterrent drug disulfiram (Antabuse). (Alcohol can also

Visit Us at TNP.com

increase the chance of liver damage with niacin. See below for more on this.)

Aside from flushing, people taking niacin may experience other uncomfortable side effects. About 1 in 4 people taking niacin experience nausea or intestinal problems. Dry skin, rash, numbness and tingling of the arms and legs, insomnia, and low blood pressure have all been reported at lower, but still significant rates of incidence—around 5 to 10% of people taking niacin. The research on niacin tends to show that higher dosages produce more side effects.

Liver Problems

Besides the relatively minor side effects described above, niacin can cause one serious health problem: liver inflammation or even outright damage. This problem occurs chiefly with the prescription-only slow-release form of niacin, although it can occur with any type of niacin.

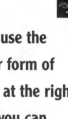

If you use the proper form of niacin at the right dose, you can often avoid side effects and other health risks.

In one major study comparing slow-release niacin to the ordinary form, 52% of the slow-release group had to drop out because of elevated liver enzymes, which are a sign of liver damage, compared to none in the immediate-release group.[11]

The good news is that liver problems are generally mild and go away when you stop taking niacin. However, there have been four reports of liver failure associated with niacin use; all of these people took slow-release niacin.[12] One person required a liver transplant. Liver toxicity has appeared after as little as 1 week of therapy and up to as long as 48 months after therapy began.

Flu-like symptoms can be a warning sign of liver problems. These include malaise, fatigue, weakness, sleepiness, appetite loss, nausea, vomiting, stomach pain, and dark urine.[13] However, it is better to catch liver problems early, which can only be accomplished through regular blood tests.

Warning: Because niacin can be hard on the liver, anyone with active liver disease (such as hepatitis or cirrhosis) or a history of liver disease should avoid niacin completely. The effects could be potentially fatal. People who drink large amounts of alcohol on a regular basis should avoid niacin for the same reason.

Drug Interactions

Niacin should not be taken along with statin drugs (see chapter 6, The Statin Family: Powerful Medications with Few Side Effects). The combination can cause *rhabdomyolysis,* a condition of severe muscle destruction that can lead to kidney failure. For this reason, it also may not be advisable to combine niacin with red yeast rice, a natural treatment (see chapter 3) that contains substances in the statin family. As mentioned previously, disulfiram (Antabuse), a drug used to treat alcoholism, may intensify the flushing side effect of niacin, so avoid this combination.

> **If you are taking a statin drug, consult your doctor before you take any niacin supplement.**

Warning: Do not combine niacin with any other cholesterol-lowering drugs, especially statin drugs. Serious reactions may occur.

Other Warnings

Niacin is an effective treatment for high cholesterol in people with diabetes. However, it may raise blood-sugar levels and make control of the diabetes more difficult.[14] Other studies have not found this effect, however, so you should consult your doctor for the latest information.

I don't recommend niacin for people with gout or a tendency to form kidney stones. Niacin can interfere with the body's excretion of uric acid. High levels of uric acid in the blood can worsen gout or cause kidney stones to form. Niacin has never been shown to cause either of these diseases in healthy people, but it seems prudent for those who already suffer from gout or kidney stones to avoid niacin.

Many types of intestinal complaints have been attributed to niacin use, so people with peptic ulcers or other intestinal complaints (such as heartburn, nausea, or vomiting) should stay away from niacin.

Warning: As mentioned above, adding niacin to an already compromised liver could be potentially fatal. As with many herbs, medications, and nutritional supplements, niacin's safety for pregnant and nursing women is unknown.

Should Children Take Niacin?

High cholesterol is sometimes found in children who have a genetic predisposition toward it (see chapter 1, What Causes Atherosclerosis?). One study examined niacin as a cholesterol-lowering treatment for children.[15] This study showed that niacin was effective in reducing total cholesterol and LDL ("bad") cholesterol. However, 76% of the children experienced side effects, and 29% had elevated liver enzymes, indicating that their livers had been irritated or damaged. Based on this study, I don't recommend niacin for children except as a last resort and under the close supervision of a pediatrician.

Lifestyle Changes

Most physicians would agree that sufficient exercise and healthful diet and lifestyle choices are the cornerstones of good health. This chapter will give you information about specific changes in your diet, exercise habits, and lifestyle that can lower your cholesterol and protect you against cardiovascular disease.

The National Cholesterol Education Program (a government-funded group of scientists) recommends that you try changing your diet, exercise, and lifestyle habits before you consider drug or herbal therapy. If you have mild to moderately high cholesterol, you might not need any further treatment to bring your cholesterol to a desirable level. Even if you do end up needing to use a drug or natural supplement to reduce your cholesterol level, you'll get better, longer-lasting results if you combine the treatment with a healthful diet and exercise routine, and above all, if you give up smoking and excessive drinking. In fact, the benefits of a healthful diet and lifestyle go far beyond merely reducing your cholesterol level. They can improve your health in a number of ways, protecting you not only from heart disease, but from a number of other serious health risks as well.

Before making changes in your diet, I recommend that you consult a health-care practitioner who is knowledgeable about nutrition (such as a nutritionist, naturopathic physician, or a medical doctor with nutritional training). Also, consult your physician before starting any exercise program. Your doctor can advise you on which exercise program may be the best for you.

Quit Smoking

The best advice about smoking is the bluntest: Stop as soon as you can. Good things start to happen in your body soon after you quit. Cigarette smoking is such a widespread and signifi-cant risk factor for heart disease that the U.S. Surgeon General has called it "the most important of the known modifiable risk factors for coronary heart disease in the United States."

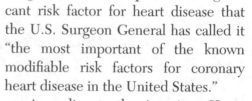

According to the U.S. Surgeon General, cigarette smoking is "the most important of the known modifiable risk factors for coronary heart disease in the United States."

According to the American Heart Association, a smoker has more than twice a nonsmoker's risk for having a heart attack. Cigarette smoking is the risk factor most associated with sudden cardiac death. Smokers who suffer a heart attack are more likely to die and die suddenly (within 1 hour) than non-smokers. Evidence also suggests that passive smoking (chronic exposure to secondhand tobacco smoke) may in-crease the risk of heart disease.

I wish I could tell you that it's easy to quit smoking. I *can* tell you that it's worth the trouble. If you want to quit smoking, consult your doctor for advice and help.

Better Nutrition

Most people are pressed for time. With busy work schedules, taking care of the kids, and trying to spend time with friends and family, they feel they don't have time to cook. Eating on the run, skipping meals, and fast food seem to be the norm in our society. As a result, the quality of our meals has declined.

This isn't to say that you can't lead an active life and still have a good diet. In fact, it's easier than you might think. Above all, you can improve your diet greatly just by becoming more aware of the food you eat—what's in it and what it does in your body. Even if you never eat at home, you can eat a more healthful diet just by knowing more about the health effects of ordinary foods.

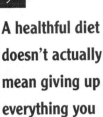

A healthful diet doesn't actually mean giving up everything you enjoy.

On the subject of making dietary changes, people often ask, "Does this mean I can't eat anything good?" or "Can I still eat my favorite dish?" Making dietary changes is *not* the same as going on a diet. This may mean shifting one's diet as a whole in a generally healthier direction.

For example, someone who eats a lot of steak could try switching some of the time to grilled salmon. The fat you get from beef is saturated fat that will tend to raise your cholesterol, but the fat in salmon (omega-3 fatty acids and other polyunsaturated fats) may actually lower your cholesterol.

A healthful diet doesn't actually mean giving up everything you enjoy. There are specific scientific reasons for the recommendations to consume less saturated fat, meat, and alcohol, and more whole grains, legumes, fresh fruits, and vegetables. With practice, you can achieve a healthier diet without sacrificing pleasure.

Reduce Saturated Fats and Increase Unsaturated Fats

We get two kinds of fat from our food. *Saturated fats* are found in almost anything that contains fat, but are highest in animal products including red meat, whole milk, butter, and lard, and in some vegetable sources, such as palm or coconut oils and vegetable shortening. Because of their chemical structure, saturated fats tend to be opaque or solid at room temperature.

Unsaturated fats are either *monounsaturated,* which means they have only one double bond between carbon molecules, or *polyunsaturated,* which means they have more than one double bond between carbon molecules. Monounsaturated fats are found in large quantities in olive oil, canola oil, and other nut oils. Polyunsaturated fats are found in corn oil, safflower oil, soybean oil, and cold-water fish such as salmon. Both types of unsaturated fats tend to be liquid at room temperature.

> **For healthier cooking, use monounsaturated fats such as olive oil and canola oil.**

Saturated fats seem to be a major culprit in raising cholesterol levels. The unsaturated fats, by contrast, actually seem to lower cholesterol levels.[1,2] Monounsaturated fats may be best for cooking, because they don't break down easily with heat. For healthier cooking, use monounsaturated fats such as olive oil and canola oil. Polyunsaturated fats can be more easily transformed into unhealthy *lipid peroxides* at high temperatures.

A 1997 review of studies tried to determine how dietary fatty acids and cholesterol affected cholesterol in the blood.[3] The authors found that replacing saturated fat with either polyunsaturated fat or monounsaturated fat led to a decline in cholesterol. Reducing dietary cholesterol also resulted in a drop in blood cholesterol. The combined effect from the dietary changes used in these trials was about a 10 to 15% decrease in total cholesterol. This is a pretty large reduction. Changing the fats in your diet alone can reduce your cholesterol at least as effectively as taking garlic!

Simply reducing the total amount of fat in your diet can help too. In a 1998 review, 19 controlled studies were evaluated, and the analysis of these trials found that restricting the amount of fat in your diet (to less than 30% of total calories) lowered cholesterol by an average of 6%.[4] However, it's interesting to note that changing the *type* of fat in the diet is more effective than reducing the *total amount* of fat.

Cut Back on Trans Fatty Acids

Although margarine was introduced on the market as being healthier than butter, this may not be true. Margarine is high in unusual fats called trans fatty acids. These substances seem to *raise* total cholesterol; even worse, they seem to raise LDL ("bad") cholesterol and reduce HDL ("good") cholesterol.[5,6] Any food that contains "hydrogenated" or "partially hydrogenated" oils also contains these unhealthy fats. However, this is a rapidly evolving subject of research. A study performed at the Mayo Clinic suggested that a form of margarine from Finland does lower cholesterol due to the presence of a special constituent made from wood pulp called *stanol ester*. Currently, two brands of this new cholesterol-lowering margarine are widely available. However, the long-term effects of these products have not been studied and are unknown.

Increase Your Intake of Fiber

It has been well documented that a lowfat, high-fiber diet can reduce the risk of certain cancers, particularly colon cancer. Fiber may also lower your cholesterol level.

Dietary fiber is primarily derived from the cell walls of plants. It is especially high in whole, unprocessed grains, fruits, and vegetables, and in legumes such as dried beans and lentils. Fiber is important in many functions of the intestinal tract, including digestion and the excretion of wastes. Fiber also removes bile acids from the gut, and thus has a mild cholesterol-lowering effect. One class of cholesterol-lowering medication—the resin drugs—works on the same principle (see chapter 6).

There are two kinds of fiber: *soluble fiber*, which swells up and holds water; and *insoluble fiber*, which does not. Soluble fiber is found in *psyllium* (a plant grown primarily in Asia and India), apples, and oat bran. Insoluble fiber consists mainly of *cellulose*, which is the main constituent of the cell walls in most plants. Most plant-based foods contain insoluble fiber, but wheat bran and flaxseeds are particularly good sources of it. Insoluble fiber seems to provide the best protection against colon cancer, but when it comes to lowering cholesterol, soluble fiber seems to be more effective. One double-blind placebo-controlled study found that psyllium husks reduced LDL ("bad") cholesterol by 5% over 24 weeks.[7] Although the decrease in LDL was modest, every little bit counts, especially when the treatment is safe.

It appears that adding soluble fiber to your diet can lower cholesterol by about 5 to 15%, depending on the type and amount of fiber used.

Other forms of fiber may be more effective. A double-blind placebo-controlled study found that oat bran reduced total cholesterol by 13% more and LDL ("bad") cholesterol by 17% more than placebo. In the same study, rice bran—a soluble fiber—did almost as well.[8] Other studies have found similar results.[9,10]

Based on these studies, it appears that adding soluble fiber to your diet can lower cholesterol by about 5 to 15%, depending on the type and amount of fiber used. Soluble fiber is found in almost all fruits, vegetables, and legumes. If you take a fiber supplement, the recommended dose is also about 10 grams daily, with plenty of water.

Exercise, Exercise, Exercise

It has been clearly established over the years that regular exercise can help improve your lipid profile. Based on some studies, it appears that aerobic exercise can lower cholesterol by about 10 to 15%, as well as improve levels of LDL, HDL, and triglycerides.[11,12] Exercise also has many other health benefits: It can help you lose weight; lower your blood pressure; decrease stress; and increase your strength, flexibility, and energy. There is also evidence that regular exercise can help you live longer.[13,14]

The best types of exercise for reducing cholesterol are aerobic exercises such as walking, jogging, bicycling, swimming, or any other activity that gets your heart rate up for a sustained period of time. Aerobic exercise is different from muscle-building activity such as weight lifting. While building muscle also seems to offer health benefits, it is primarily aerobic exercise that reduces cholesterol levels.

The best thing about aerobic exercise is that it is easy to do and doesn't cost a lot of money. You don't have to buy an expensive treadmill or exercise bike. Simply taking brisk walks can be quite beneficial. The key to any successful exercise program is *consistency.* If you only exercise once in a blue moon, you're not likely to see results. But even a modest amount of exercise several times a week can give you results over time.

To get the maximum benefit from aerobic exercise, you need to continue the activity for a sustained time period with moderate intensity. In other words, you should feel like you're working pretty hard, without feeling strained or exhausted. For example, if you choose to go walking, a slow stroll is not as beneficial as walking at a quick pace. However, it is very important that you don't overwork yourself, especially if you're just starting an exercise program. Start slowly and build up your stamina over time.

Remember, the effects of exercise are cumulative. If you can stay motivated to do it consistently, you are more likely to improve your cholesterol level.

While no one seems to agree on an exact program for everyone, it appears that moderate aerobic exercise three to five times per week for 15 to 30 minutes can help lower your cholesterol. The trick is finding a type of exercise that is fun for you. Torturing yourself will probably be counterproductive,

Erik's Story

Erik, 39, works for a large computer company and puts in long days. In an employee health screening, he learned that his cholesterol was 237 mg/dL. His doctor recommended that he go on a statin drug; however, Erik was opposed to using a drug at that point, and wanted to try a more natural approach first.

Regarding his diet, Erick said, "I get to work around 7 a.m. and usually start my morning with a doughnut and coffee—the company provides them for free. I'm at my desk all morning, and then someone usually goes to a local fast-food restaurant and gets lunch for all of us. By the time I get off work around 9 p.m., I'm too tired to cook, so I pick up a sandwich or burger on my way home."

It was apparent that Erik's job was interfering with his ability to get regular exercise and eat well. He admitted that it was possible for him

because you won't keep it up. Choose an activity that you enjoy and that you can manage to do regularly. Also, try to be patient. Many people get frustrated when first starting a program, because the results aren't immediately obvious. Expect that it will take some time to build up your endurance, especially if you haven't exercised in a while. The same may be true for your cholesterol. Remember, the effects of exercise are cumulative, which means that if you can stay motivated to do it consistently, you are more likely to have your cholesterol drop and stay down.

Before starting any exercise program, consult your doctor to see whether you have any medical conditions that might limit your choice of exercise. Your physician can also suggest specific activities that might be better for you.

Warning: If at any point during exercise, you begin to experience chest pain, dizziness, or breathlessness, discontinue the activity and consult your physician immediately.

to take a lunch break if he wanted. He agreed to take a 15-minute walk around the grounds of his office and to bring his meals to work—including more fruits and vegetables in his lunches.

After 2 months, Erik's cholesterol had started to take a plunge. It had decreased from 237 mg/dL to 212 mg/dL. He said he was still eating quite a few burgers and fried foods, and he was going to cut back on those even more.

After 1 more month, his cholesterol was down to a normal value of 193 mg/dL. He had virtually stopped his "burger run" after work, and he was eating more vegetables, fruits, and grains. It took him 3 months to make the necessary changes in his diet and lifestyle, but he never had to use a drug or supplement to control his cholesterol.

Alcohol: Only in Moderation

Studies suggest that moderate drinking of beer, wine, or spirits can actually reduce the risk of heart disease.[15,16] However, the American Heart Association generally discourages drinking because of the dangers associated with excessive use, such as alcoholism, hypertension, obesity, stroke, liver disease, and cancer, as well as the danger of automobile accidents (from driving while intoxicated) or other accidents (falling down, for instance).

In one study, the equivalent of two drinks a day of any kind of alcohol lowered the incidence of heart disease compared to not drinking.[17] But consuming more than two drinks a day resulted in a higher risk of heart attack and stroke. In this study, red wine showed stronger effects against heart disease than other alcoholic beverages. The study's author suggested that this might be because red wine contains flavonoids, which may help reduce cholesterol levels. Flavonoids are antioxidant substances found in many fruits and vegetables. You don't need to drink wine to get them in your diet.

Changing Your Overall Lifestyle Really Does Work!

The bottom-line question for all of these lifestyle changes is: Will they really reduce my risk of death or disease related to atherosclerosis? The answer is yes. It appears that a healthful lifestyle may not only lower your cholesterol but also reverse atherosclerosis.

> **It appears that a healthful lifestyle cannot only lower your cholesterol but even reverse atherosclerosis.**

The Lifestyle Heart Trial, a study spearheaded by Dr. Dean Ornish, demonstrated that lifestyle changes can reverse existing atherosclerosis.[18] This controlled study involved 48 participants with documented atherosclerosis in the arteries of their hearts. Twenty-eight participants were randomly assigned to an experimental group that ate a lowfat vegetarian diet, stopped smoking, got moderate exercise, and underwent stress management training. The other 20 individuals were asked to continue living their normal life. These participants were followed for 1 year.

At the end of the year, each person was given an angiogram—a medical test that measures blockage in the arteries. Of the participants who made the lifestyle changes, 82% had less atherosclerosis than they had at the study's outset. The average blockage of the coronary arteries in the lifestyle change group dropped from 40 to 37.8%, while the blockage in the control group increased from 42.7 to 46%.

While it's difficult to say how much each separate lifestyle change contributed to the total effect, this study seems to demonstrate that exercising, choosing to eat a healthier diet, and avoiding high-risk activities may not only prevent—but actually reverse—atherosclerosis.

Conventional Treatments for High Cholesterol

T he leading recommended treatment for high cholesterol is not a drug or an herb (see chapter 5). The National Cholesterol Education Program (a U.S. government council of doctors and scientists) recommends trying dietary and lifestyle changes before resorting to any sort of pill. Only when these fundamental approaches do not work should you use the drugs discussed in this chapter, which covers the conventional medications that can be used as a safety net.

How Effective Are Cholesterol-Lowering Drugs?

Very effective cholesterol-lowering drugs are available today. In clinical practice and in research, the "statin drugs" have been shown to lower total cholesterol by up to 35%, LDL ("bad") cholesterol by 30 to 40%, and triglycerides by 30%. They can also increase HDL ("good") cholesterol by 5 to 10%. Like all medical treatments, however, these benefits come along with some risks and side effects.

The first cholesterol-reducing "drug" was actually the vitamin niacin (vitamin B_3). It was introduced as a cholesterol-lowering agent more than 40 years ago, and it is still used today.

Niacin has been shown to improve all cholesterol measurements, and it actually reduces mortality rates (see chapter 4).

In the mid- to late-1960s, bile acid-sequestering resins and fibric acid derivatives came on the market as alternatives to niacin. Bile acid-sequestering drugs and fibric acid derivatives are fairly successful at lowering cholesterol, but have some problems that limit their clinical usefulness (see Bile Acid-Sequestering Resins: Too Many Side Effects). In 1987, the newest class of cholesterol-lowering drugs, the statin drugs, became available. This class of drugs is more effective at lowering total cholesterol and LDL than the other drugs on the market, with substantially fewer side effects. Interestingly, one natural treatment for high cholesterol—red yeast rice—contains substances in the statin family. The statin drugs are the most widely used today.

Whether or not you use a prescription medication (or take garlic, for that matter), diet and lifestyle are still very important.

The Statin Family: Powerful Medications with Few Side Effects

Statin drugs have greatly improved the treatment of high cholesterol. Drugs in this class include lovastatin (Mevacor), pravastatin (Pravachol), simvastatin (Zocor), fluvastatin (Lescol), and atorvastatin (Lipitor). They've been available in the United States for just over 10 years, somewhat longer in European countries.

Lovastatin, the first of these drugs, was introduced in 1987. It was originally isolated from a strain of the common fungus *Aspergillus tereus*. Today, lovastatin is produced synthetically. Substances very similar to lovastatin are also found in red yeast rice (see chapter 3). Other statin drugs have subsequently been

Sam's Story

Sam was a 37-year-old athlete. "It's not fair," he said. "I exercise 2 hours daily and run marathons. I'm also a vegetarian, and the only fat I get is from olive oil and canola oil. Yet my total cholesterol level is over 375. Why is the universe picking on me?"

It turned out that Sam's father had died of a heart attack at age 47. This event was partly responsible for Sam's vigorous lifestyle: He didn't want the same thing to happen to him. "Only nothing I do seems to be working," he complained.

Clearly, for Sam there was a genetic factor at work. It was probably genetics that killed his father, and the same would happen to him if he didn't successfully lower his cholesterol.

Sam's lifestyle was helping him. But because his cholesterol was so high, garlic or other natural treatments probably wouldn't have been effective. He took the cholesterol-lowering drug simvastatin, and within 2 months his total cholesterol was under 200. This tremendous improvement was a testament not only to the medication, but to Sam's lifestyle. He had done his part; adding a medication carried him the rest of the way.

introduced by competing pharmaceutical companies. All of them appear to function similarly.

Statin drugs work by interfering with the body's normal production of cholesterol. In the liver and other tissues, an enzyme called HMG-CoA reductase controls the rate at which the body manufactures cholesterol. When your cholesterol level is low, your body produces more HMG-CoA reductase, which in turn creates more cholesterol. When your cholesterol levels are where they should be, HMG-CoA production is turned off. In this way, your body has a built-in mechanism, like a thermostat, to keep cholesterol levels in the optimal range, neither too high nor too low. When your cholesterol levels are too high it is because this built-in function is not working properly.

The statin drugs directly affect the body's "thermostat" by inhibiting the action of HMG-CoA reductase. (Interestingly, garlic may work the same way, and red yeast rice almost certainly does. See chapters 2 and 3.) When you take a drug or herb that inhibits HMG-CoA reductase, you inhibit the body's ability to produce more cholesterol. The net result is that cholesterol levels decline. Of all the cholesterol-lowering drugs, this class is by far the most effective. Not only can these medications improve cholesterol levels significantly, they can also save lives.

Because the statins are drugs that you may take for a lifetime, any possibility of increased risk of cancer is worrisome.

The first major study of a statin drug (lovastatin) found that it decreased total cholesterol by 22%, and LDL ("bad") cholesterol by 31%. HDL ("good") cholesterol increased by 5%.[1] Not only did lovastatin produce positive results; it did far better than placebo. Lovastatin also acted relatively quickly. After only 2 weeks, the group taking lovastatin was doing noticeably better than the placebo group.

The Scandinavian Simvastatin Survival Study, published in 1995, was a double-blind placebo-controlled trial that evaluated 4,444 participants with a history of either chest pain or previous heart attack.[2] Half the group received simvastatin while the other half received placebo that looked just like the drug. Researchers followed both groups for just over 5 years.

This study confirmed the earlier research. Total cholesterol fell by 25%, and LDL ("bad") cholesterol dropped 35%, while HDL ("good") cholesterol went up 8%. Furthermore, this study added a very important finding: There was a whopping 42% decrease in death from heart disease in the group taking simvastatin, and a 30% decrease in death from all causes. While

12% of the participants in the placebo group died during the course of the study, only 8% of the people in the simvastatin group died. Thus, this study showed that taking a statin drug can increase long-term survival.

This type of study is important because it shows that the drug is doing what we want it to do. Although we know that high cholesterol is associated with increased death from heart disease, this does not guarantee that a drug that lowers cholesterol will actually reduce the risk of death from heart disease. Drugs have many effects, and it is always possible that unrecognized bad effects may outweigh the good ones. This study showed that simvastatin produces an effect that is highly beneficial overall.

All of the statin drugs are effective at lowering cholesterol. However, as with most classes of medications, people react to the statin drugs in individual ways. For example, a person who may not see any cholesterol reduction with lovastatin can be switched to pravastatin or simvastatin and see substantial results. It is not clear why this phenomenon occurs, but it is typical of all medical treatments, including herbs. (A new area of drug research, called *pharmacogenetics*, is beginning to help us understand why this may be. It appears that different responses to drugs can sometimes be accounted for by genetic differences in the people taking the drugs.)

Safety Issues

Besides their effectiveness, another major advantage to statin drugs is that they have a low incidence of side effects. The most common problem is headache, but it occurs in less than 2% of those who take these medications. Also, a small number of people have allergic reactions to these drugs. Other occasional side effects of statin drugs include abdominal pain, constipation, diarrhea, nausea, headaches, dizziness, skin rash, blurred vision, and joint pain; however, these side effects go away when the statin drug use ends.

There were some early reports that these drugs caused opacification, or clouding of the lens in the eye. But larger studies have since shown that this is not true. However, there are some significant safety concerns when using these medications: liver toxicity, muscle and kidney damage, increased cancer risk, and CoQ_{10} depletion.

Liver Toxicity

A more serious potential side effect of statin drugs is liver toxicity. In laboratory tests, about 1 to 2% of those who take these drugs show signs of significant liver inflammation. Physicians evaluate the health of the liver by measuring the level of enzymes that normally leak out of the liver. When the liver cells become damaged, these enzymes leak out at an increased rate, raising levels of these enzymes in the blood. For this reason, you will hear the description "elevated liver enzymes" to describe evidence of liver problems.

In one large study of pravastatin, about 1% of the treated group showed a threefold elevation in liver enzymes. This is not as bad as it sounds, however, because there was a similar elevation in 0.75% of the placebo group, showing that in many cases, the elevation of enzymes was due to something other than the treatment.[3] For example, even modest use of alcohol elevates liver enzymes. Still, your liver is so important that current recommendations suggest that if you take a statin drug, you need to check your liver enzymes after 6 weeks of therapy. Fortunately, liver enzymes generally return to normal soon after the drug is stopped.

Muscle and Kidney Damage

A rare but very serious side effect of statin drugs is an inflammation of the muscles that causes severe muscle damage. Even worse, the products of dying muscle can destroy the kidney. This rare and little-understood side effect has mostly been seen when statin drugs are combined with certain other medications, such as niacin, erythromycin, cyclosporine, or fibrate drugs. Your physician or pharmacist can advise you whether it is safe to combine statins with other medications you may be taking.

Do Statin Drugs Increase Cancer Risk?

Probably the biggest question regarding statin drugs is lingering concerns that they may increase the risk of cancer. Laboratory tests on mice have found a slight but significant increase in the incidence of certain cancers in female mice (but not in male mice). Other studies have found an increased cancer incidence in both male and female rodents at doses 3 to 33 times higher than the usual human dose, and still other animal studies have found that HMG-CoA reductase inhibitors cause mutation in cells, the usual first step in the development of cancer.

None of the studies on humans have found a significantly increased incidence of cancer, but the longest human study lasted only 5 years, and the drugs themselves have been in use for only a decade or so. Since this is a drug that you may take for a lifetime, any possibility of increased risk of cancer is worrisome.

Some respected medical authorities have interpreted the animal research findings to mean that the statin drugs should not even be on the market. Others point to the fairly dramatic evidence of reduction in death from heart disease, and feel that the benefits outweigh the risk.

There is no simple answer to this controversy. Many of these issues can only be answered over time with careful examination of the magnitude of the risks and benefits of using these drugs. I recommend that you consult closely with your physician to decide whether these medications are appropriate for you.

Coenzyme Q_{10} Depletion

An important but rarely recognized side effect of taking a statin drug is the depletion of a naturally occurring substance called coenzyme Q_{10} (CoQ_{10}).[4,5] It appears that the very same process that inhibits HMG-CoA reductase also reduces CoQ_{10} production. This side effect is "silent," because there are no obvious symptoms that occur when CoQ_{10} levels drop. It's not entirely clear whether CoQ_{10} depletion causes any health problems, but the result probably isn't that great for you.

CoQ_{10} is a nutrient that the body needs to transform food into energy. It is found in almost every cell of the body. CoQ_{10} is also a powerful antioxidant. CoQ_{10} can be taken as a supplement, and it has been used to treat a variety of health conditions, especially those related to heart disease.

Although we don't know for sure what the consequences of CoQ_{10} depletion may be, it may be wise to take 30 mg daily as insurance. CoQ_{10} appears to be a very safe supplement. The maximum safe dosage in young children, pregnant or nursing women, or those with severe liver or kidney disease has not been determined. (For more information on CoQ_{10}, see *The Natural Pharmacist: Natural Health Bible.*)

Warning: If you have congestive heart failure, you should not suddenly *stop* taking CoQ_{10}, as doing so might cause your symptoms to temporarily worsen.

Bile Acid-Sequestering Resins: Too Many Side Effects

Cholestyramine (Questran) and colestipol (Colestid) are members of one of the oldest categories of drugs used to lower cholesterol, the bile acid-sequestering resins. Although effective, these drugs have fallen out of favor because of their relatively high incidence of side effects. Cholestyramine and colestipol work in an interesting, roundabout way.

Bile acids are formed in the liver and used to break down fatty foods. They contain considerable quantities of cholesterol. Normally, after bile acids have done their work on a fatty meal, the body reabsorbs them and the cholesterol they contain. Bile acid-sequestering resins work by binding to numerous substances, including bile acids. As these drugs move through the intestinal tract, they act like a strong magnet attracting bile acids and forming a combined molecule that cannot be reabsorbed. This cholesterol is then lost to the body.

In order to make more bile acids, the liver has to get some spare cholesterol from somewhere. One of its main sources is cholesterol floating about in the blood. The net result of this complex chain of events is that cholesterol levels in the blood are reduced.

These drugs typically reduce total cholesterol by about 10%, and decrease LDL ("bad") cholesterol by up to 20%, while raising HDL ("good") cholesterol by 3 to 8%.

Unfortunately, bile acid-sequestering resins pose several problems. They are taken in the form of powder, which is mixed with liquid and drunk like a milk shake. This "resin milk shake" tastes terrible to most people. I recall one man describing his experience as "trying to drink sand in rotten milk." Some people try to mix the powder in juice or applesauce to mask the taste and texture, but you won't find too many people rushing to the pharmacy to fill this prescription as a taste treat.

Another problem is gastrointestinal side effects such as bloating, diarrhea, flatulence, nausea, vomiting, and constipation. While not dangerous, these side effects can be extremely unpleasant. Furthermore, along with cholesterol, these resins also remove fat-soluble vitamins from the body, such as vitamins A, D, E, and K. If they are used for a long period of time, genuine deficiencies can develop. One of the most serious possible consequences is an excess tendency to bleed due to vitamin K deficiency.

Resins can also bind a variety of medications that we'd rather keep within our bodies, such as penicillin, digoxin (a heart medication), propranolol (taken for high blood pressure), thyroid hormone, and warfarin (taken to prevent blood clotting). People using resin drugs are advised to take any other medication at least 1 hour before or 4 hours after taking the resin.

Fibric Acid Derivatives: Better for Treating High Triglyceride Levels

Triglycerides can also increase the risk of heart disease, although they are not as dangerous as cholesterol. Still, if triglyceride levels are high enough, they can cause problems. The fibric acid drugs are most useful for people with mildly elevated cholesterol but very high triglyceride levels.

This class of drugs includes gemfibrozil (Lopid) and clofibrate (Atromid-S). We do not really know how they work. However, there is no question that they do work. A 5-year double-blind placebo-controlled study of 4,081 men found that gemfibrozil reduced triglycerides by 35%, but only reduced cholesterol by 8%. Over this 5-year period, there was an overall decrease of 34% in mortality from coronary heart disease.[6]

However, other studies have not shown any reduction in death from cardiovascular disease, and a few have even shown an overall *increase* as high as 44% in the rate of death due to conditions other than cardiovascular diseases, including cancer, complications following gallbladder removal, and *pancreatitis* (inflammation of the pancreas).[7]

Fibric acid drugs also cause significant digestive upset in as many as 34% of people who take them.[8] Rare and more severe side effects include gallbladder disease, liver inflammation, muscle inflammation, kidney damage, and bone marrow injury. Finally, there is a concern that these drugs may increase the incidence of cancer, even more so than the statin drugs.

Putting It All Together

For your easy reference, this chapter contains a brief summary of key information contained in this book. Please refer to earlier chapters for more comprehensive information, including a detailed discussion of safety issues.

There is reasonably strong evidence showing that garlic is an effective treatment for reducing mild to moderately elevated cholesterol levels. Studies suggest that taking garlic can reduce total cholesterol by an average of 10 to 12%, while also reducing triglycerides and LDL ("bad") cholesterol. Besides lowering cholesterol, garlic appears to have other positive benefits related to atherosclerosis: reducing blood pressure, preventing platelets from sticking to each other, promoting the breakdown of blood clots, and protecting cells from free-radical damage.

There are many forms of garlic, but garlic powder standardized to contain 1.3% alliin has the most research behind it. The recommended dose of such garlic powder is 600 to 900 mg daily. Aged garlic may also be helpful, taken at doses of 1 to 7.2 grams daily. In general, garlic is a safe treatment with few side effects, except for a garlicky odor on the body and/or breath. Aged garlic in particular has been proven very safe.

Warning: Garlic should not be combined with prescription blood thinners such as warfarin (Coumadin) or heparin.

Garlic is most effective for people whose blood cholesterol levels are mildly to moderately high. If your cholesterol level is above 300 mg/dL, garlic undoubtedly won't be effective enough for you if used alone. If you can't bring your cholesterol down with natural methods, it's important that you don't rule out using medications. The risks of heart disease and strokes far outweigh the risks of drugs.

Other Natural Treatments for Cholesterol

Besides garlic, other herbs and supplements also seem to have a cholesterol-lowering effect. High-dose niacin is a well-established treatment for high cholesterol. There is strong evidence that 500 mg of niacin taken 3 times daily can lower cholesterol up to 15%. "Flushing" is a common side effect.

Warning: Medical supervision is necessary when using high-dose niacin treatment to reduce cholesterol levels.

Red yeast rice is another promising new treatment for lowering cholesterol. Early studies suggest that 600 mg twice daily may lower cholesterol up to 30%.

Preliminary evidence also suggests that 500 mg of the herbal extract gugulipid taken 3 times a day may be helpful in lowering cholesterol 10 to 15%.

Pantethine may reduce cholesterol when taken at a dose of 300 mg 3 times a day and may have an even more dramatic impact on lowering triglycerides.

Finally, tocotrienols at a dose of 200 mg a day may also offer some benefits.

Other supplements, such as vitamin C, essential fatty acids, glycosaminoglycans, and L-carnitine may be helpful, but the research remains weak, and in some cases, contradictory.

Last but not least, diet and lifestyle can reduce cholesterol levels, reverse atherosclerosis, and protect you from a variety of illnesses and health risks. If you want to reduce your risk of heart disease, the single most important change you can make in your lifestyle is to quit smoking. A diet low in saturated (animal) fats and trans fatty acids (margarine), and high in polyunsaturated and monounsaturated fats, can significantly reduce your cholesterol level.

Soy foods may also help reduce cholesterol levels. According to the FDA, you need to get about 25 grams of soy protein daily to lower your cholesterol.

A regular aerobic exercise program can also help improve your cholesterol levels and your overall health.

Notes

Atherosclerosis and High Cholesterol

1. Robbins S, Cotran R, Kumar V. *Robbins pathologic basis of disease.* 5th ed. Philadelphia: Saunders; 1994.

2. Strong JP, et al. Early lesions of atherosclerosis in childhood and youth: natural history and risk factors. *J Am Coll Nutr.* 1992;11:51S–54S.

3. Strong JP. The natural history of atherosclerosis in childhood. *Ann NY Acad Sci.* 1991;623:9–15.

4. Schaefer EJ, et al. Lipoprotein(a) levels and risk of coronary heart disease in men. The Lipid Research Clinics Coronary Primary Prevention Trial. *JAMA.* 1994;271:999–1003.

5. Scanu AM, Fless GM. Lipoprotein(a): a genetic risk factor for premature coronary heart disease. *JAMA.* 1992;267:3326–3329.

Garlic for High Cholesterol

1. Steinmetz KA, et al. Vegetables, fruit and colon cancer in the Iowa Women's Health Study. *Am J Epidemiol.* 1994;139(1):1–15.

2. Ernst E. Can allium vegetables prevent cancer? *Phytomedicine.* 1997;4(1):79–83.

3. Schulz V, et al. *Rational phytotherapy.* 3rd ed. New York: Springer-Verlag; 1998:114.

4. Agarwal KC, et al. Therapeutic actions of garlic constituents. *Med Res Rev.* 1996;1:111–124.

5. Mader FH. Treatment of hyperlipidemia with garlic-powder tablets. Evidence from the German Association of General Practitioners' multicentric placebo-controlled double-blind study. *Arzneimittelforschung Drug Res*. 1990;40(10):1111–1116.

6. Greenberg RP, et al. A meta-analysis of fluoxetine outcome in the treatment of depression. *J Nerv Ment Dis*. 1994;182(10):547–551.

7. Jain AK, et al. Can garlic reduce levels of serum lipids? A controlled clinical study. *Am J Med*. 1993;94:632–635.

8. Silagy CA, Neil HA. Garlic as a lipid lowering agent—a meta-analysis. *J R Coll Physicians Lond*. 1994;28(1):39–45.

9. Warshafsky S, et al. Effect of garlic on total serum cholesterol: A meta-analysis. *Ann Intern Med*. 1993;119:599–605.

10. Steiner M, et al. A double-blind crossover study in moderately hypercholesterolemic men that compared the effect of aged garlic extract and placebo administration on blood lipids. *Am J Clin Nutr*. 1996;64:866–870.

11. De A Santos OS, Johns RA. Effects of garlic powder and garlic oil preparations on blood lipids, blood pressure and well-being. *Br J Clin Res*. 1995;6:91–100.

12. Reuter HD, et al. *Allium sativum* and *Allium ursinum:* Part 2. Pharmacology and Medicinal Application. *Phytomedicine*. 1995;2:73–91.

13. Berthold HK, et al. Effect of a garlic oil preparation on serum lipoproteins and cholesterol metabolism: a randomized controlled trial. *JAMA*1998;279(23):1900–1902.

14. Neil HA, et al. Garlic powder in the treatment of moderate hyperlipidemia: a controlled trial and meta-analysis. *J R Coll Physicians Lond*. 1996;30(4):329–34.

15. Isaacsohn JL, et al. Garlic powder and plasma lipids and lipoproteins: a multicenter, randomized, placebo-controlled trial. *Arch Intern Med*. 1998;158(11):1189–1194.

16. Simons LA, et al. On the effect of garlic on plasma lipids and lipoproteins in mild hypercholesterolemia. *Atherosclerosis*. 1995;113:219–225.

17. Holzgartner H, et al. Comparison of the efficacy and tolerance of a garlic preparation vs. bezafibrate. *Arzneimittelforschung Drug Res*. 1992;42(12):1473–1477.

18. Lachmann G, et al. Untersuchungen zur pharmakokinetik der mit 35S markierten knoblauchinhaltsstoffe alliin, allicin und vinyldithiine. *Arzneimittelforschung Drug Res*. 1994;44:734–743.

19. Qureshi AA, et al. Inhibition of cholesterol and fatty acid biosynthesis in liver enzymes and chicken hepatocytes by polar fractions of garlic. *Lipids*. 1983;18(5):343–348.

20. Gebhardt, R. Multiple inhibitory effects of garlic extracts on cholesterol biosynthesis in hepatocytes. *Lipids*. 1993;28(7):613–619.

21. Gebhardt R, Beck H. Differential inhibitory effects of garlic-derived organosulfur compounds on cholesterol biosynthesis in primary rat hepatocyte cultures. *Lipids*. 1996;31(12):1269–1276.

22. Yeh Y, Yeh S. Garlic reduces plasma lipids by inhibiting hepatic cholesterol and triacylglycerol synthesis. *Lipids*. 1994;29(3):189–193.

23. Sendl A, et al. Inhibition of cholesterol synthesis in vitro by extracts and isolated compounds prepared from garlic and wild garlic. *Atherosclerosis*. 1992;94:79–85.

24. Gebhardt R, Beck H. Differential inhibitory effects of garlic-derived organosulfur compounds on cholesterol biosynthesis in primary rat hepatocyte cultures. *Lipids*. 1996;31(12):1269–1276.

25. Eilat S, et al. Alteration of lipid profile in hyperlipidemic rabbits by allicin, an active constituent of garlic. *Coron Artery Dis*. 1995;6:985–990.

26. Chandorkar AG, Jain PK. Analysis of hypotensive action of *Allium sativum*. *Indian J Physiol Pharmacol*. 1973;17:132–133.

27. Foushee DB, et al. Garlic as a natural agent for the treatment of hypertension: a preliminary report. *Cytobios*. 1982;34:135–136, 145–152.

28. Auer W, et al. Hypertension and hyperlipidemia: garlic helps in mild cases. *Br J Clin Pract Suppl*. 1990;69:3–6.

29. Silagy CA, Neil HA. A meta-analysis of the effect of garlic on blood pressure. *J Hypertens*. 1994;12:463–468.

30. Das I, et al. Potent activation of nitric oxide synthase by garlic: a basis for its therapeutic applications. *Curr Med Res Opin*. 1995;13(5):257–263.

31. Pedraza-Chaverri J, et al. Garlic prevents hypertension induced by chronic inhibition of nitric oxide synthesis. *Life Sci*. 1998;62(6):71–77.

32. Dirsch VM, et al. Effect of allicin and ajoene, two compounds of garlic, on inducible nitric oxide synthase. *Atherosclerosis*. 1998;139(2):333–339.

33. Siegel G, et al. Potassium channel activation in vascular smooth muscle. *Adv Exp Med Biol*. 1992;311:53–72.

34. Siegel G, et al. Potassium channel activation, hyperpolarization, and vascular relaxation. *Z Kardiol*. 1991;80(suppl 7):9–24.

35. Orekhov AN, Grunwald J. Effects of garlic on atherosclerosis. *Nutrition*. 1997;13(7–8):656–663.

36. Breithaupt-Grogler K, et al. Protective effect of chronic garlic intake on elastic properties of aorta in the elderly. *Circulation*. 1997;96(8):2649–2655.

37. Das I, et al. Potent activation of nitric oxide synthase by garlic: a basis for its therapeutic applications. *Curr Med Res Opin*. 1995;13(5):257–263.

38. Steiner M, Lin RS. Changes in platelet function and susceptibility of lipoproteins to oxidation associated with administration of aged garlic extract. *J Cardiovasc Pharmacol*. 1998;31(6):904–908.

39. Kiesewetter H, et al. Effect of garlic on thrombocyte aggregation, microcirculation, and other risk factors. *Int J Clin Pharmacol Ther Toxicol*. 1991;29(4):151–155.

40. Kleijnen J, et al. Garlic, onions and cardiovascular risk factors. A review of the evidence from human experiments with emphasis on commercially available preparations. *Br J Pharmac*. 1989;28:535–544.

41. Reuter HD, et al. *Allium sativum* and *Allium ursinum*: Part 2. Pharmacology and Medicinal Application. *Phytomedicine*. 1995;2:73–91.

42. Reuter HD, et al. *Allium sativum* and *Allium ursinum*: Part 2. Pharmacology and Medicinal Application. *Phytomedicine.* 1995;2:73–91.

43. Reuter HD, et al. *Allium sativum* and *Allium ursinum*: Part 2. Pharmacology and Medicinal Application. *Phytomedicine.* 1995;2:73–91.

44. Chutani SK, Bordia A. The effect of fried versus raw garlic on fibrinolytic activity in man. *Atherosclerosis.* 1981;38:417–421.

45. Yamasaki T, Lau BH. Garlic compounds protect vascular endothelial cells from oxidant injury. *Nippon Yakurigaku Zasshi.* 1997;110(suppl 1):138–141.

46. Lewin G, Popov I. Antioxidant effects of aqueous garlic extract. 2nd. Communication: Inhibition of the Cu2+-initiated oxidation of low density lipoproteins. *Arzneimittelforschung Drug Res.* 1994;44(5):604–607.

47. Ide N, Lau BH. Garlic compounds protect vascular endothelial cells from oxidized low density lipoprotein-induced injury. *J Pharm Pharmacol.* 1997;49(9):908–911.

48. Horie T, et al. Identified diallyl polysulfides from an aged garlic extract which protects the membranes from lipid peroxidation. *Planta Med.* 1992;58(5):468–469.

49. Phelps S, Harris WS. Garlic supplementation and lipoprotein susceptibility *Lipids.* 1993;28(5):475–477.

50. Prasad K, et al. Antioxidant activity of allicin, an active principle in garlic. *Mol Cell Biochem.* 1995;148:183–189.

51. Imai J, et al. Antioxidant and radical scavenging effects of aged garlic extract and its constituents. *Planta Med.* 1994;60(5):417–420.

52. Yamasaki T, Lau BH. Garlic compounds protect vascular endothelial cells from oxidant injury. *Nippon Yakurigaku Zasshi.* 1997;110(suppl 1):138–141.

53. Bordia A, et al. Knoblauch und koronare herzkrankheit: Wirkungen einer dreijahrigen behandlung mit knob-lauchextrakt auf die reinfarkt und mortalitatsrate [Garlic and coronary heart disease: results of a three year treatment with garlic extract on reinfarction

and mortality rate]. *Deutsche Apotheker Ztg.* 1989;28(suppl15): 16–17.

54. Yeh Y, et al. Cholesterol lowering effects of aged garlic extract supplementation on free-living hypochol esterolemic men consuming habitual diets. *J Am Coll Nutr.* 1995;13:545.

55. Lau BHS, et al. Effect of an odor-modified garlic preparation on blood lipids. *Nutr Res.* 1987;7:139–149.

56. Steiner M, et al. A double blind crossover study in moderately hypercholesterolemic men comparing the effect of aged garlic extract and placebo administration on blood lipids and platelet function. *Shinyaku To Rinsho.* 1996;45(3):456–466.

57. Lawson LD, et al. Identification and HPLC quantitation of the sulfides and dialk(en)yl thiosulfinates in commercial garlic products. *Planta Med.* 1991;57:363–370.

58. Lau BHS, et al. Effect of an odor-modified garlic preparation on blood lipids. *Nutr Res.* 1987;7:139–149.

59. Bordia A. Effect of garlic on blood lipids in patients with coronary heart disease. *Am J Clin Nutr.* 1981;34(10):2100–2103.

60. Vorberg G, Schneider B. Therapy with garlic: results of a placebo-controlled, double-blind study. *Br J Clin Pract Suppl.* 1990;69:7–11.

61. Schulz V, et al. *Rational phytotherapy.* 3rd ed. New York: Springer-Verlag; 1998:121–122.

62. Mader FH. Treatment of hyperlipidemia with garlic-powder tablets. Evidence from the German Association of General Practitioners' multicentric placebo-controlled double-blind study. *Arzneimittelforschung Drug Res.* 1990;40(10):1111–1116.

63. Schulz V, et al. *Rational phytotherapy.* 3rd ed. New York: Springer-Verlag; 1998.

64. Burden AD, et al. Garlic-induced systemic contact dermatitis. *Contact Dermatitis.* 1994;30(5):299–300.

65. McFadden JP, et al. Allergic contact dermatitis from garlic. *Contact Dermatitis.* 1992;27(5):333–334.

66. Lembo G, et al. Allergic contact dermatitis due to garlic *(Allium sativum). Contact Dermatitis.* 1991;25(5):330–331.

67. Garty BZ. Garlic burns. *Pediatrics.* 1993;91(3):658–659.

68. Holzgartner H, et al. Comparison of the efficacy and tolerance of a garlic preparation vs. bezafibrate. *Arzneimittelforschung Drug Res.* 1992;42(12):1473–1477.

69. Ernst E. Can Allium vegetables prevent cancer? *Phytomedicine.* 1997;4(1):79–83.

70. Steinmetz KA, et al. Vegetables, fruit, and colon cancer in the Iowa Women's Health Study. *Am J Epidemiol.* 1994;139(1):1–15.

71. Dausch JG, Nixon DW. Garlic: A review of its relationship to malignant disease. *Prev Med.* 1990;19:346–361.

72. Sumiyoshi H, et al. Chronic toxicity test of garlic extract in rats [in Japanese]. *J Toxicol Sci.* 1984;9:61–75.

73. Yoshida S, et al. Mutagenicity and cytotoxicity tests of garlic [in Japanese]. *J Toxicol Sci.* 1984;9:77–86.

74. German K, et al. Garlic and the risk of TURP bleeding. *Br J Urol.* 1995;76:518.

75. Abdullah T, et al. Enhancement of natural killer cell activity in AIDS with garlic. *Onkologie.* 1989;21:52–53.

76. Kandil O, et al. Garlic and the immune system in humans: its effects on natural killer cells. *Fed Proc.* 1987;46(3):441.

Other Supplements for High Cholesterol

1. Heber D, et al. Cholesterol-lowering effects of a proprietary Chinese red-yeast-rice dietary supplement. *Am J Clin Nutr.* 1999;69:231–236.

2. Chang J, et al. Elderly patients with primary hyperlipidemia benefited from treatment with a Monacus purpureus rice preparation: A placebo-controlled, double-blind clinical trial. *American Heart Association's 39th Annual Conference on Cardiovascular Disease Epidemiology and Prevention.* Orlando, Florida; March, 1999.

3. Chang M. Cholestin: *Healthcare professional product guide.* Simi Valley, CA: Pharmanex; 1998:1–6.

4. Singh RB, et al. Hypolipidemic and antioxidant effects of *Commiphora mukul* as an adjunct to dietary therapy in patients with

hypercholesterolemia. *Cardiovasc Drugs Ther.* 1994;8(4):659–664.

5. Nityanand S, et al. Clinical trials with gugulipid: A new hypolipidemic agent. *J Assoc Phys India.* 1989;37(5):323–328.

6. Verma SK, Bordia A. Effect of Commiphora mukul (gum guggulu) in patients of hyperlipidemia with special reference to HDL cholesterol. *Indian J Med Res.* 1988;87:356–360.

7. Agarwal RC, et al. Clinical trial of gugulipid—a new hypolipidemic agent of plant origin in primary hyperlipidemia. *Indian J Med Res.* 1986;84:626–634.

8. Singh V, et al. Stimulation of low density lipoprotein receptor activity in liver membrane of guggulsterone treated rats. *Pharmacol Res.* 1990;22(1):37–44.

9. *Gugulipid—six months toxicity data in rats and beagles.* Central Drug Research Institute; 1982: Dossier 8–58.

10. *Gugulipid—Phase II clinical data.* Central Drug Research Institute; 1981: Dossier 5–8.

11. *Gugulipid—six months toxicity data in rats and beagles.* Central Drug Research Institute; 1982: Dossier 8–58.

12. Gaddi A, et al. Controlled evaluation of pantethine, a natural hypolipidemic compound, in patients with different forms of hyperlipoproteinemia. *Atherosclerosis.* 1984;50:73–83.

13. Angelico M, et al. Improvement in serum lipid profile in hyperlipoproteinemic patients after the treatment with pantethine: a cross-over, double blind trial versus placebo. *Curr Ther Res.* 1983;33(6):1091–1097.

14. Coronel F, et al. Treatment of hyperlipidemia in diabetic patients on dialysis with a physiological substance. *Am J Nephrol.* 1991;11(1):32–36.

15. Donati C, et al. Pantethine, diabetes mellitus and atherosclerosis. Clinical study of 1,045 patients [in Italian]. *Clin Ther.* 1989;128(6):411–422.

16. Cighetti G, et al. Modulation of HMG-CoA reductase activity by pantetheine/pantethine. *Biochem Biophys Acta.* 1988;963(2):389–393.

17. Arsenio L, et al. Effectiveness of long-term treatment with pantethine in patients with dyslipidemia. *Clin Ther*. 1986;8(5):537–545.

18. Howard PA, Meyers DG. Effect of vitamin C on plasma lipids. *Ann Pharmacother*. 1995;29:1129–1136.

19. Gerster H. No contribution of ascorbic acid to renal calcium oxalate stones. *Ann Nutr Metab*. 1997;41(5):269–282.

20. Qureshi AA, et al. Novel tocotrienols of rice bran modulate cardiovascular disease risk parameters of hypercholesterolemic humans. *J Nutr Biochem*. 1997;8:290–298.

21. Parker RA, et al. Tocotrienols regulate cholesterol production in mammalian cells by post-transcriptional suppression of 3-hydroxy-3-methylglutaryl-Coenzyme A reductase. *J Biol Chem*. 1993;268(15):11230–11238.

22. Tomeo AC, et al. Antioxidant effects of tocotrienols in patients with hyperlipidemia and carotid stenosis. *Lipids*. 1995;12:1179–1183.

23. Anderson JW, Johnstone BM, Cook-Newell ME. Meta-analysis of the effects of soy protein intake on serum lipids. *N Engl J Med*. 1995;333:276–282.

24. Kromhout D, et al. Alcohol, fish, fiber and antioxidant vitamins intake do not explain population differences in coronary heart disease mortality. *Int J Epidemiol*. 1996;25:753–759.

25. Dyerberg J. n-3 Fatty Acids and coronary artery disease. potentials and problems. *Omega-3. Lipoproteins and Atherosclerosis*. 1996;27:251–258.

26. Harris WS. n-3 Fatty acids and serum lipoproteins: human studies. *Am J Clin Nutr*. 1997;65(suppl):1645S–1654S.

27. Dyerberg J. n-3 Fatty Acids and coronary artery disease. potentials and problems. *Omega-3. Lipoproteins and Atherosclerosis*. 1996;27:251–258.

28. Prichard BN, et al. Fish oils and cardiovascular disease. *BMJ*. 1995;310:819–820.

29. Stone NJ. From the Nutrition Committee of the American Heart Association. Fish consumption, fish oil, lipids, and coronary heart disease. *Am J Clin Nutr*. 1997;65:1083–1086.

Notes

30. Harris WS. Dietary fish oil and blood lipids. *Curr Opin Lipidol*. 1996;7:3–7.

31. Harris WS. n-3 Fatty acids and serum lipoproteins: human studies. *Am J Clin Nutr*. 1997;65(suppl):1645S–1654S.

32. Laurora G, et al. Control of the progress of arteriosclerosis in high risk subjects treated with mesoglycan. Measuring the intima media [in Italian]. *Minerva Cardioangiol*. 1998;46:41–47.

33. Tanganelli P, et al. Updating on in-vivo and in-vitro effects of heparin and other glycosaminoglycans (mesoglycan) on arterial endothelium: a morphometrical study. *Int J Tissue React*. 1992;14(3):149–153.

34. Morrison LM, Enrick L. Coronary heart disease: Reduction of death rate by chondroitin sulfate. A *Angiology*. 1973;24(5):269–287.

35. Nakazawa K, Murata K. The therapeutic effect of chondroitin polysulphate in elderly atherosclerotic patients. *J Int Med Res*. 1978;6(3):217–225.

36. Saba P, et al. Hypolipidemic effect of mesoglycan in hyperlipidemic patients. *Curr Ther Res*. 1986;40:761–768.

37. Davini P, et al. Controlled study on L-carnitine therapeutic efficacy in post-infarction. *Drugs Exp Clin Res*. 1992;18(8):355–365.

38. Bell L, et al. Cholesterol-lowering effects of calcium carbonate in patients with mild to moderate hypercholesterolemia. *Arch Intern Med*. 1992;152:2441–2444.

39. Oosthuizen W, et al. Lecithin has no effect on serum lipoprotein, plasma fibrinogen and macro molecular protein complex levels in hyperlipidaemic men in a double-blind controlled study. *Eur J Clin Nutr*. 1998;52(6):419–424.

Niacin and High Cholesterol

1. Canner PI, et al. Fifteen year mortality in coronary drug project patients: long term benefit with niacin. *J Am Coll Cardiol*. 1986;8:1245–1255.

2. McKenney JM, et al. A comparison of the efficacy and toxic effects of sustained- vs. immediate-release niacin in hypercholesterolemic patients. *JAMA*. 1994;271:672-677.

3. Christensen AN, et al. Nicotinic acid treatment of hyper cholesterolemia. *JAMA.* 1961;177:546–550.

4. Knopp RH, et al. Contrasting effects of unmodified and time-release forms of niacin on lipoproteins in hyperlipidemia subjects: clues to mechanism of action of niacin. *Metabolism.* 1995;34:642–650.

5. Superko HR, Krauss RM. Differential effects of nicotinic acid in subjects with different LDL subclass patterns. *Atherosclerosis.* 1992;95:69–76.

6. Smith CM, Reynard AM. *Essentials of Pharmacology.* Philadelphia: W.B. Saunders; 1995:306.

7. Jin FY, et al. Niacin decreases removal of high-density lipoprotein apolipoprotein A-1 but not cholesterol ester by Hep G2 cells. Implication for reverse cholesterol transport *Arterioscler Thromb Vasc Biol.* October 17, 1997;(10):2020–2028.

8. Alderman JD, et al. Effect of two aspirin pretreatment regimens on niacin-induced cutaneous reactions. *J Gen Intern Med.* 1989;12:591–596.

9. Jungnickel PW, et al. Effect of two aspirin pretreatment regimens on niacin-induced cutaneous reactions. *J Gen Intern Med.* 1997;12:591–596.

10. Head KA. Inositol hexaniacinate: A safer alternative to niacin. *Alt Med Rev.* 1996;1(3):176–184.

11. McKenney JM, et al. A comparison of the efficacy and toxic effects of sustained- vs. immediate-release niacin in hypercholesterolemic patients. *JAMA.* 1994;271:672–677.

12. Head KA. Inositol hexaniacinate: A safer alternative to niacin. *Alt Med Rev.* 1996;1(3):176–184.

13. Clementz GL, Holmes AW. Nicotinic acid-induced fulminant hepatic failure. *J Clin Gastroenterol.* 1987;9:582–584.

14. Schwartz ML. Severe reversible hyperglycemia as a consequence of niacin therapy. *Arch Intern Med.* 1993;153(17):2050–2052.

15. Colletti RB, et al. Niacin treatment of hypercholesterolemia in children. *Pediatrics.* 1993;92(1):78–82.

Lifestyle Changes

1. Truswell AS, Choudhury N. Monounsaturated oils do not all have the same effect on plasma cholesterol. *Eur J Clin Nutr*. 1998;52(5):312–315.

2. Kris-Etherton PM, Yu S. Individual fatty acid effects on plasma lipids and lipoproteins: human studies. *Am J Clin Nutr*. 1997;65(suppl 5):1628S–1644S.

3. Clarke R, et al. Dietary lipids and blood cholesterol: quantitative meta-analysis of metabolic ward studies. *BMJ*. January 11, 1997;(314):112–117.

4. Tang JL, et al. Systematic review of dietary intervention trials to lower total blood cholesterol in free-living subjects. *BMJ*. 1998;316:1213–1220.

5. Mensink RP, Katan MB. Effect of dietary trans fatty acids on high-density and low-density lipoprotein cholesterol levels in healthy subjects. *N Eng J Med*. August 16, 1990;323(7):439–445.

6. Sundram K, et al. Trans (elaidic) fatty acids adversely affect the lipoprotein profile relative to specific saturated fatty an humans. *J Nutr*. March 1997;127(3):514–520S.

7. Davidson MH, et al. Long-term effects of consuming foods containing psyllium seed husk on serum lipids in subjects with hypercholesterolemia. *Am J Clin Nutr*. March 1998;67(3):367–376.

8. Gerhardt AL, Gallo NB. Full-fat rice bran and oat bran similarly reduce hypercholesterolemia in humans. *J Nutr*. 1998;128(5):865–869.

9. Goel V, et al. Cholesterol lowering effects of rhubarb stalk fiber in hypercholesterolemic men. *J Am Coll Nutr*. December 1997;16(6):600–604.

10. Sprecher DL, et al. Efficacy of psyllium in reducing serum cholesterol levels in hypercholesterolemic patients on high or low-fat diets. *Ann Intern Med*. 1993;119(7):545–554.

11. Schuit AJ, et al. The effect of six months training on weight, body fatness and serum lipids in apparently healthy elderly Dutch men and women. *Int J Obes Relat Metab Disord*. September 1998;22(9):847–853.

12. Dengel DR, et al. Improvements in blood pressure, glucose metabolism and lipoprotein lipids after aerobic exercise plus weight loss in obese, hypertensive middle-aged men. *Metabolism.* September 1998;47(9):1075–1082.

13. Erikssen G, et al. Changes in physical fitness and changes in mortality. *Lancet.* 1998;352:759–762.

14. Leon AS, et al. Leisure time physical activity and the 16-year risks of mortality from coronary heart disease and all-causes in the multiple risk factor intervention trial (MRFIT). *Int J Sports Med.* July 1997;18(suppl 3):S208–S215.

15. Klatsky AL, et al. Alcohol and mortality. *Ann Intern Med.* 1992;117:646–654.

16. Steinberg D, et al. Alcohol and atherosclerosis. *Ann Intern Med.* 1991;114:967–976.

17. Constant J. Alcohol, ischemic heart disease, and the French paradox. *Coron Artery Dis.* October 1997;8(10):645–649.

18. Ornish D, et al. Can lifestyle changes reverse coronary heart disease? *Lancet.* 1990;336:129–133.

Conventional Treatments for High Cholesterol

1. *Physicians' desk reference.* 52nd ed. Montvale, NJ: Medical Economics; 1998:938.

2. Kjekshus J, Pedersen TR. Reducing the risk of coronary events: evidence from the Scandanavian simvastatin survival study. *Am J Cardiol.* 1995;76(9):64C–68C.

3. *Physicians' desk reference.* 52nd ed. Montvale, NJ: Medical Economics; 1998:938.

4. Ghirlanda G, et al. Evidence of plasma CoQ_{10}-lowering effect by HMG-CoA reductase inhibitors: a double-blind, placebo-controlled study. *J Clin Pharmacol.* 1993;33(3):226–229.

5. Bargossi AM, et al. Exogenous CoQ_{10} supplementation prevents plasma ubiquinone reduction induced by HMG-CoA reductase inhibitors. *Mol Aspects Med.* 1994;15(suppl):187–193.

6. Frick MH, et al. Helsinki heart study: primary-prevention trial with gemfibrozil in middle-aged men with dyslipidemia. *N Eng J Med*. 1987;317:1237–1245.

7. *Physicians' desk reference*. 52nd ed. Montvale, NJ: Medical Economics; 1998:938.

8. *Physicians' desk reference*. 52nd ed. Montvale, NJ: Medical Economics; 1998:938.

Index

A

Acetaminophen in Extra Strength Tylenol, 39

Aerobic exercise, 97

Aged garlic, 111
  advantages of, 48–49
  preparation of, 44–45
  studies of, 41
  toxicity of, 60

Ajoene, 28
  in garlic oil, 47

Alcohol use
  flavonoids and, 99–100
  moderation in, 99–100
  and niacin, 87–88

Allergic reactions
  to garlic, 52
  to statin drugs, 105

Allicin, 13, 28
  in aged garlic, 45
  in garlic oil, 47
  and HMG-CoA reductase, 28

Alliin, 13
  in aged garlic, 24–25, 45
  in garlic oil, 47
  mechanics of, 28
  standardized herbal extracts for, 41

Allinase, 13
  in garlic powder, 42–43

Allium sativum. See Garlic

Alpha-tocopherol. *See* Vitamin E

American Heart Association
  on alcohol use, 99

on cholesterol levels, 5
  on cigarette smoking, 92
  Step I diet, 67

Amino acids
  in garlic, 14
  L-carnitine, 79
  tryptophan, 81

Anaphylaxis, 52

Angina
  atherosclerosis and, 1

Angiograms, 100

Antabuse and niacin, 87–88, 89

Anti-depressant, garlic as, 51

Antioxidants, 4

Aortic glycosaminoglycans (GAGs), 78–79, 112
  scientific evidence for, 79

Apples, 95

Arteries. *See also* Atherosclerosis
  lumen, 5
  pulse wave velocity measurement, 34

Ascorbic acid. *See* Vitamin C

Aspergillus tereus, 102

Aspirin
  garlic and, 35–36, 61
  with niacin, 85

Atherosclerosis, 1–10
  causes of, 3–5
  diagnosis of, 9–10
  garlic and, 29, 33–35
  notes on, 115
  response to injury hypothesis, 4

Atherosclerosis *(continued)*
  risk factors, 2–3
  tocotrienols and, 76
  triglycerides and, 7
Atorvastatin, 102
Atromid-S, 110
Ayurvedic medicine, gugulipid in, 69

B

Bezafibrate and garlic, 27, 57–58
Bicycling, 97
Bile, 6
Bile acid-sequestering resins, 102,
    108–109
  drug interactions with, 109
  safety issues of, 108–109
Blood
  atherosclerosis and, 4
  garlic and, 60–61
Blood clotting and thinning
  aortic glycosaminoglycans
    (GAGs) and, 79
  garlic and, 18, 35–36, 61
Brammer, Debra, 80
Breastfeeding women. *See* Nursing
    women
Breath, garlic odor and, 54–55
Bruit, 9
Bubonic plague, garlic and, 17
Bulbils of garlic, 12
Burns from garlic, 57

C

Calcium and cholesterol, 79–80
Cancer. *See also* Colon cancer
  cholesterol-lowering drugs and,
    58–59
  fiber intake and, 95
  fibric acid derivatives and, 110
  garlic and, 58–59
  red yeast rice and, 69
  statin drugs and, 107
Cardiac risk factors, 8
Cardiovascular disease. *See* Heart
    disease

Carnitine, 79, 112
Catheterization for atherosclerosis,
    10
Cellulose, 95
Chang, Joseph, 67
Childbirth, garlic and, 60–61
Children
  gugulipid for, 71
  niacin for, 90
China, garlic use in, 16
Cholesterol. *See also* Garlic; HDL
    (high density lipoprotein);
    LDL (low density lipoprotein);
    Niacin
  aortic glycosaminoglycans
    (GAGs) and, 78–79
  calcium and, 79–80
  combination therapy for, 80
  defined, 6
  determining levels of, 7–8
  gugulipid, 69–71
  L-carnitine and, 79
  lecithin and, 80
  lifestyle changes and, 91–100
  link to high cholesterol, 5
  omega-3 fatty acids and, 78
  red yeast rice, 65–69
  soy and, 77–78
  tocotrienols, 75–77
  vitamin C, 73–75
Cholesterol-lowering drugs. *See*
    Statin drugs
Cholestin, red yeast rice and, 66–67
Cholestyramine, 108
Cigarette smoking, 92
  atherosclerosis and, 3
Cirrhosis and niacin, 89
Clofibrate, 110
  gugulipid compared, 70
Clot-dissolving drugs, 36
Coenzyme Q_{10} and statin drugs,
    107–108
Colds, vitamin C and, 74
Colestid, 108
Colestipol, 108

Colic
  garlic and, 64
  vitamin C and, 75
Colon cancer
  fiber intake and, 95
  garlic and, 59
  insoluble fiber and, 95–96
Combination therapy for choles-
    terol, 80
Commiphoral mukus. See Gugulipid
Commission E
  on aged garlic, 45
  on dosages of garlic, 38–39
  use of garlic, 18
Complicated plaque, 5
Conenzyme A (CoA), 71–72
Contraindications to garlic, 51–53
Conventional treatments. *See also*
    Statin drugs
  garlic compared, 26–27, 57–59
  for high cholesterol, 101–110
  notes on, 127–128
Coumadin
  bile acid sequestering resins and,
    109
  garlic and, 53, 61
CT scans for atherosclerosis, 10
Cyclosporine
  red yeast rice and, 69
  statin drugs and, 106

D
Da suan, 16
Depression
  garlic and, 51
Dermatitis, garlic and, 57
Diabetes
  garlic and, 62–63
  niacin and, 89
  omega-3 fatty acids and, 78
  pantethine and, 72
Diagnosis of atherosclerosis, 9–10
Diallyl disulfide, 28
Diallyl trisulfide, 28
Diastolic blood pressure, 30

Diet
  fats, reducing amount of,
    93–94
  fiber intake, increasing, 95–96
  garlic in, 46–47
  improving nutrition, 92–96
  niacin in, 83
  trans fatty acids, reducing, 95
Digoxin, bile acid-sequestering
    resins and, 109
Dioscorides, 15, 16
Disulfiram and niacin, 87–88,
    89
Doppler studies, 10
Dosages
  for garlic, 38–39
  for gugulipid, 71
  for niacin, 84–85
  for pantethine, 73
  for red yeast rice, 68
  for tocotrienols, 76–77
  for vitamin C, 74
Double-blind placebo-controlled
    studies, 20
Drug interactions
  with bile acid-sequestering resins,
    109
  with garlic, 61–63
  with gugulipid, 71
  with niacin, 89
  with pantethine, 73
  with red yeast rice, 69
  with vitamin C, 75
Drug monitoring studies, 56

E
Ebers Codex, 15
E-guggulsterone, 71
Egyptians, garlic use by, 14–15
Endothelium, injury to, 4
Erythromycin
  red yeast rice and, 69
  statin drugs and, 106
Estrogen, cholesterol and, 6
EWL-60-S test, 51

Exercise, 96–99, 112
Extra Strength Tylenol, aceta-
    minophen in, 39

F

Fats, reducing amounts of, 93–94
Feverfew, garlic and, 53
Fiber intake, increasing, 95–96
Fibrate drugs
    red yeast rice and, 69
    statin drugs and, 106
Fibric acid derivatives, 102,
    109–110
Fibrin, 36
Fibrinolysis, 36
Fibrous plaque, 5
Fish oil. *See* Omega-3 fatty acids
Flavonoids
    alcohol use and, 99–100
    in garlic, 14
    red yeast rice fermentation and,
        66
Flaxseeds, 95
Flush-free niacin, 86
Flushing and niacin, 85, 87, 112
Fluvastatin, 102
14-alpha demethylase, 29
Four Thieves Vinegar, 17, 44–45
Framingham Heart Study, 2–3
Free radicals, 4

G

Gaby, Alan, 75
Galen, 15, 16
Gallbladder disease, fibric acid de-
    rivatives and, 110
Garlic, 9, 11–12, 111–112. *See also*
    Aged garlic; Alliin; Garlic oil;
    Garlic powder
    aged garlic, 24–25
    allergic reactions to, 52
    allicin in, 13–14
    in ancient world, 14–15
    as antioxidant, 36–37
    and atherosclerosis, 29, 33–35
    bezafibrate compared, 57–58

blood and, 60–61
blood clotting and, 35–36
bulbils, 12
bulbs of, 11
burns from, 57
cloves of, 11
combination therapy with, 80
contraindications to, 51–53
conventional medications com-
    pared, 26–27, 57–59
cooking with fresh garlic, 46–47
cultivating, 11–12
defined, 13–14
dermatitis and, 57
diabetes and, 62–63
dilating blood vessels, 32–33
dosages of, 38–39
drug interactions with, 61–63
drug monitoring studies, 56
drying methods, 42–43
eating fresh garlic, 46–47
expectations from, 49–51
fried garlic, 41
HDL (high density lipoprotein)
    and, 23–24
heart disease deaths and, 37–38
high blood pressure and, 30–33
historical use of, 14–18
and HMG-CoA reductase, 28
LDL (low density lipoprotein)
    and, 23–24
long-term risk, 58–59, 63–64
Mader study on, 21–23
mechanics of, 27–29
meta-analysis of, 24
in modern medicine, 18–19
mood improvements, 51
name, meaning of, 12–13
notes on, 115–121
odor, problems with, 54–55
organ transplants and, 62
pemphigus and, 62
preparations, types of, 42–48
preparing fresh garlic, 46–47
raw garlic, side effects from,
    56–57

safety issues, 54–60
scientific evidence for, 19–29
standardized herbal extract of, 30–42
temporary setbacks from, 49–50
toxicity of, 59–60
type of garlic, 41, 48–49
whole person, treating the, 53
Garlic oil, 25
  preparation of, 47–48
  studies of, 41
Garlic powder, 111
  allinase in, 42–43
  bezafibrate, comparison to, 27
  dosages for, 39
  drying methods, 42–43
  high blood pressure and, 30–31
  odorless products, 55
  preparation of, 42–44
  studies of, 25–26, 41
Garlic vinegar, 49
Gemfibrozil, 110
Genotoxicity, 60
Germany. *See also* Commission E
  garlic in, 11
  Mader study on garlic, 21–23
Ginkgo
  garlic and, 53, 61
  studies on, 19
Glucose as irritant in blood, 4
Greeks, garlic use by, 15–16
Guggulsterones, 71
Gugulipid, 69–71, 112
  clofibrate compared, 70
  dosages for, 71
  drug interactions with, 71
  notes on, 121–124
  safety issues, 71
  scientific evidence for, 69–71

H

HDL (high density lipoprotein), 6
  bile acid-sequestering resins and, 109
  cardiac risk factors, 8
  exercise and, 96

garlic and, 23–24
garlic powder and, 26
gugulipid and, 70
lecithin and, 80
levels of, 8
niacin and, 82–83
red yeast rice and, 66–68
statin drugs and, 101
trans fatty acids and, 95
Heart attacks
  clot-dissolving drugs, 36
  garlic and, 38
Heart disease
  alcohol use and, 99
  cardiac risk factors, 8
  coenzyme Q_{10} and, 108
  fibric acid derivatives and, 110
  garlic and deaths from, 37–38
  lipoprotein(a) and, 7
Hebrews, garlic use by, 15
Hemochromatosis, vitamin C and, 75
Hemophilia, garlic and, 60
Hemostasis, garlic and, 35–36
Heparin, garlic and, 61
Hepatitis and niacin, 89
Herbal treatments. *See* Garlic
High blood pressure
  garlic and, 30–33
  omega-3 fatty acids and, 78
Hippocrates, 15–16
  whole person, treating the, 53
History of garlic use, 14–18
HMG-CoA reductase
  garlic and, 28
  mevinolin and, 66
  pantethine inhibiting, 72–73
  statin drugs and, 103–104
  tocotrienols inhibiting, 76
Homocysteine
  as irritant in blood, 4
  omega-3 fatty acids and, 78
Hong Qu, 65
Hypertension. *See* High blood pressure
Hypoglycemia, 62–63

I

Inositol hexaniacinate, 86
Insoluble fiber, 95
Intermittent claudication, 2
Iron and vitamin C, 75

J

Jogging, 97
Journal of the American Medical Association garlic oil study, 25

K

Kidneys, 106
   gugulipid and, 71
   niacin and, 89–90
   pantethine and, 73
   red yeast rice and, 69
   tocotrienols and, 77
   vitamin C and, 75

L

L-carnitine, 79, 112
LD$_{50}$ (lethal doses in 50%), 59
LDL (low density lipoprotein), 6, 111
   atherosclerosis and, 4
   bile acid-sequestering resins and, 109
   cardiac risk factors, 8
   exercise and, 96
   free radicals and, 37
   garlic and, 23–24
   garlic powder and, 26
   gugulipid and, 70
   lecithin and, 80
   levels of, 7–8
   lipoprotein (a), 6–7
   omega-3 fatty acids and, 78
   pantethine and, 72
   psyllium husks and, 96
   red yeast rice and, 66–68
   soy and, 77–78
   statin drugs and, 101
   tocotrienols and, 76
   trans fatty acids and, 95
Lecithin and cholesterol, 80
Lescol, 102

Lifestyle changes, 91–100. *See also* Diet
   notes on, 126–127
   significance of, 100
Lifestyle Heart Trial, 100
Lipid peroxides, 94
Lipid profile, 7
Lipids, 6
   in garlic, 14
Lipitor, 102
Lipoprotein(a), 6–7
   niacin and, 83
Lipoproteins, 6–7. *See also* HDL (high density lipoprotein); LDL (low density lipoprotein)
Liver
   bile acid-sequestering resins and, 108–109
   gugulipid and, 71
   inositol hexaniacinate and, 86
   niacin and, 85, 88–89
   pantethine and, 73
   red yeast rice and, 69
   slow-release niacin and, 88
   statin drugs and toxicity, 106
   tocotrienols and, 77
Lopid, 110
Lovastatin, 102, 104
   red yeast rice dosage compared, 68
Lumen of artery, 5

M

Macrophages, 4
Mader, F. H., 22
Mader study on garlic, 21–23
Margarine, 95
Meta-analysis
   garlic, 31–32
   of garlic, 24
   of vitamin C and cholesterol, 74
Mevacor, 102, 104
Mevinolin, 66
Middle Ages, garlic in, 16
Minerals in garlic, 14
Monascus purpureus, 65
Monounsaturated fats, 94

Mukul myrrh tree. *See* Gugulipid
Muscles
   niacin and, 89
   red yeast rice and, 69
   statin drugs and, 106
Mutagenicity, 60

N

Natural killer (NK) cells, 62
Natural treatments. *See also* Garlic
Nausea, garlic and, 56
Neil, Andrew, 30–31
Niacin, 81–90, 101–102, 112
   alcohol use and, 87–88
   for children, 90
   in diet, 83
   dosages of, 84–85
   drug interactions, 89
   flushing and, 85, 87, 112
   inositol hexaniacinate, 86
   liver problems and, 85, 88–89
   mechanics of, 84
   notes on, 121–124, 125–126
   and red yeast rice, 69, 89
   safety issues of, 86–89
   scientific evidence for, 82–83
   slow-release niacin, 86
   statin drugs and, 89, 106
   types of, 85–86
Niacinamide, 86
Notes, 115–128
Nursing women
   garlic and, 64
   pantethine for, 73
   tocotrienols in, 77
   vitamin C and, 75
Nutrition. *See* Diet

O

Oat bran, 95, 96
Occult blood tests, 75
Odor, garlic and, 54–55
Omega-3 fatty acids
   cholesterol and, 78
   notes on, 121–124
   scientific evidence for, 78

Opacification, 105–106
Organ transplants, garlic and, 62
Ornish, Dean, 100

P

Palm oil. *See* Tocotrienols
Pancreatitis, fibric acid derivatives
   and, 110
Pantethine, 71–73, 112
   dosages of, 73
   drug interactions with, 73
   notes on, 121–124
   safety issues, 73
   scientific evidence for, 72–73
Pemphigus, 62
Penicillin, bile acid-sequestering
   resins and, 109
Pentoxifyline, garlic and, 61
Pharmacogenetics, 105
Placebo effect, 20
Placebos, side effects from, 56
Plaque, 1
   complicated plaque, 5
   fibrous plaque, 5
Platelets in atherosclerosis, 4
Pliny the Elder, 15
Polyunstaurated fats, 94
Poor Man's Treacle, 16
Pravachol, 102, 105
Pravastatin, 102, 105
Pregnancy
   garlic and, 60, 64
   gugulipid and, 71
   pantethine during, 73
   tocotrienols in, 77
   vitamin C and, 75
Progesterone, cholesterol and, 6
Propranolol, bile acid sequestering
   resins and, 109
Prostaglandins, aspirin and, 85
Prostate
   TURP surgery, garlic and, 60–61
Proteins in garlic, 14
Psyllium, 95
Pulse wave velocity measurement,
   34

Q
Questran, 108

R
Recommended dietary allowance
    (RDA) of niacin, 83
Red yeast rice, 65–69, 112
    Cholestin compared, 66–67
    dosage for, 68
    drug interactions with, 69
    niacin and, 69, 89
    notes on, 121–124
    safety issues, 68–69
    scientific evidence for, 66–68
    statin drugs and, 69
    toxicity, 68
Rhabdomyolysis, 89
Rice bran oil. *See* Tocotrienols

S
Safety issues
    of bile acid-sequestering resins,
        108–109
    of garlic, 54–60
    of gugulipid, 71
    of niacin, 86–89
    of omega-3 fatty acids, 78
    of pantethine, 73
    of red yeast rice, 68–69
    of statin drugs, 105–108
    of tocotrienols, 77
    of vitamin C, 74
St. John's wort
    studies on, 19
Saturated fats, reducing, 93–94
Scandinavian Simvastatin Survival
        Study, 104
Scurvy, 73
Side effects. *See* Safety issues
Silagy, Christopher, 30–31
Simvastatin, 102, 103, 104–105
Slow-release niacin, 86
    liver problems and, 88
Soluble fiber, 95, 96

Soy foods, 77–78, 112
Spontaneous spinal epidural
        hematoma, 60
Standardized herbal extracts of gar-
        lic, 39–42
Stanol ester, 95
Statin drugs, 27, 102–108
    allergic reactions to, 105
    cancer risk and, 107
    coenzyme Q_{10} and, 107–108
    effectiveness of, 101–102
    garlic and, 51
    HMG-CoA reductase and,
        103–104
    kidney damage and, 106
    liver toxicity and, 106
    mechanics of, 103
    muscle damage and, 106
    niacin and, 82, 83, 89
    opacification, 105–106
    red yeast rice and, 69
    safety issues of, 105–108
Steroids in garlic, 14
Studies
    on aortic glycosaminoglycans
        (GAGs), 79
    on garlic, 19–29
    on gugulipid, 69–71
    on niacin, 82–83
    on omega-3 fatty acids, 78
    on pantethine, 72–73
    on red yeast rice, 66–68
    on tocotrienols, 75–76
    on vitamin C, 74
Sulfides in aged garlic, 45
Surgery, garlic and, 60–61
Swimming, 97
Systolic blood pressure, 30

T
Tempeh, 77–78
Testosterone, cholesterol and, 6
Thiol group, 62
Thrill, 9
Thrombi, 5

Thyroid hormone, bile acid-sequestering resins and, 109
Tocotrienols, 75–77
atherosclerosis and, 76
dosages for, 76–77
notes on, 121–124
safety issues, 77
scientific evidence for, 75–76
Tofu, 77–78
Toxicity
of garlic, 59–60
red yeast rice, 68
statin drugs and liver toxicity, 106
Trace elements in garlic, 14
Trans fatty acids, reducing, 95
Transient ischemic attacks (TIAs), 5
Trental, garlic and, 61
Triglycerides, 7. *See also* Garlic
exercise and, 96
fibric acid derivatives and, 109–110
garlic powder and, 26
gugulipid and, 70
L-carnitine and, 79
lecithin and, 80
levels of, 8
niacin and, 82–83
pantethine for, 71–73
red yeast rice and, 67
soy and, 77–78
statin drugs and, 101
Tryptophan, 81
TURP surgery, garlic and, 60–61

U

U. S. National Cholesterol Education Program (NCEP), 7, 101
lifestyle changes and, 91
on niacin, 82
Unsaturated fats, increasing, 93–94

V

Very VLDL (very low-density
lipoprotein), 6
Vinyldithiins, 28

in aged garlic, 45
in garlic oil, 47
Vitamin A, bile acid-sequestering
resins and, 109
Vitamin B_1, 81
Vitamin B_2, 81
Vitamin B_3. *See* Niacin
Vitamin B_6, 81. *See also* Pantethine
Vitamin C, 73–75, 112
dosages for, 74
drug interactions with, 75
niacin and, 81
safety issues, 74–75
scientific evidence for, 74
Vitamin D, bile acid-sequestering
resins and, 109
Vitamin E. *See also* Tocotrienols
bile acid-sequestering resins and,
109
cholesterol and, 6
garlic and, 53, 61
Vitamin K, bile acid-sequestering
resins and, 109

W

Walking, 97
Warfarin
bile acid sequestering resins and,
109
garlic and, 53, 61
Weight lifting, 97
Wheat bran, 95
White blood cells in atherosclerosis,
4–5
Whole person, treating the, 53
World War I, garlic in, 17
World War II, garlic in, 17

X

X-rays for atherosclerosis, 10

Z

Z-guggulsterone, 71
Zocor, 102, 103, 104–105

About the Author

Darin Ingels is a graduate of Purdue University and is a certified medical technologist. He is currently attending Bastyr University in Seattle, Washington, and is a candidate for his Doctorate of Naturopathic Medicine degree. He lives in Kirkland, Washington, with his wife, Michelle.

About the Series Editors

Steven Bratman, M.D., is medical director for TNP.com. Dr. Bratman is both a strong proponent and vocal critic of alternative treatment, and he believes that alternative medicine has both strengths and weaknesses, just like conventional medicine. This even-handed critique has made him a trusted party on both sides of the debate. He has been an expert consultant to the State of Washington Medical Board, the Colorado Board of Medical Examiners, and the Texas State Board of Medical Examiners, evaluating disciplinary cases involving alternative medicine.

His books include *The Alternative Medicine Sourcebook: A Realistic Evaluation of Alternative Healing Methods* (1997), *The Alternative Medicine Ratings Guide: An Expert Panel Ranks the Best Alternative Treatments for Over 80 Conditions* (Prima Health, 1998), the professional text *Clinical Evaluation of Medicinal Herbs and Other Therapeutic Natural Products* (Prima Health, 1999), and the following titles in THE NATURAL PHARMACIST series*: Your Complete Guide to Herbs* (Prima Health, 1999), *Your Complete Guide to Illnesses and Their Natural Remedies* (Prima Health, 1999), *Natural Health Bible* (Prima Health, 1999), and *St. John's Wort and Depression* (Prima Health, 1999).

David J. Kroll, Ph.D., is a professor of pharmacology and toxicology at the University of Colorado School of Pharmacy and a consultant for pharmacists, physicians, and alternative practitioners on the indications and cautions for herbal medicine use. He received a degree in toxicology from the Philadelphia College of Pharmacy and Science and obtained his Ph.D. from the University of Florida College of Medicine. Dr. Kroll has lectured widely and has published articles in a number of medical journals, abstracts, and newsletters.

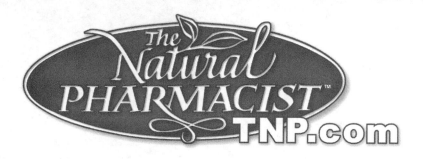

Science-Based Natural Health Information You Can Trust™

TNP.com Is:

- **Science-based**
- **Independent and unbiased**
- **Up to date**
- **Balanced—offers both positive and negative findings**
- **Integrative—includes both conventional and natural treatments**
- **M.D. and Ph.D. supervised**

From Asian Ginseng to Zinc, TNP.com cuts through the hype and tells you what is scientifically proven and what remains unknown about popular natural treatments. Setting a new, high standard of accuracy and objectivity, this Web site takes a realistic look at the herbs and supplements you hear about in the news and provides the balanced information necessary to make informed decisions about your health needs. If you want to be an informed consumer of natural products, TNP.com is the place to start.

Using TNP.com is easy, free, and private. Visit TNP.com now to get science-based natural health information you can trust!

Visit us online at www.TNP.com